To my wife

Basic Clinical Ophthalmology

Basic Clinical Ophthalmology

Calbert I. Phillips
MD (Aberd), PhD (Bristol), MSc (Manc) DPH (Ed),
FRCS (Ed and Eng), DO, FBOA (Hon)

Professor of Ophthalmology, University of Edinburgh, and
Honorary Consultant Ophthalmic Surgeon, Royal Infirmary, Edinburgh

CHURCHILL LIVINGSTONE
EDINBURGH LONDON MELBOURNE AND NEW YORK 1987

CHURCHILL LIVINGSTONE
Medical Division of Longman Group UK Limited

Distributed in the United States of America by
Churchill Livingstone Inc., 1560 Broadway, New York,
N.Y. 10036, and by associated companies, branches
and representatives throughout the world.

First published/1984 (Pitman Publishing Ltd)
    Reprinted 1985
    Reprinted 1987 (Churchill Livingstone)

ISBN 0-443-03953-4

British Library Cataloguing in Publication Data

Phillips, Calbert I.
    Basic clinical ophthalmology
1. Eye—Diseases and defects—Diagnosis
    I. Title
    617.7'15   RE75

Library of Congress Cataloging in Publication Data

Phillips, Calbert I.
    Basic clinical ophthalmology.
    1. Ophthalmology.   I. Title.   [DNLM: 1. Eye Diseases
—diagnosis.   2. Eye Diseases—therapy.
WW 140 P558b]
RE45.P48   1984   617.7   84–14727

Produced by Longman Group (FE) Ltd
Printed in Hong Kong

Contents

Preface

The main audience for which this book is being published is the undergraduate medical student in all countries, and the general practitioner. The ophthalmic resident should be familiar with all the subjects covered in the book within a few months of starting in the specialty.

We think that the ophthalmic optician, the ophthalmic nurse and the orthoptist will find many parts of it useful. Detailed advice on practical treatment and management for the non-specialist is included in most clinical problems.

Understanding is an important basis for learning, and so we have tried to present our subjects rationally, with an explanation of causation and mechanism as far as that is known. None of the concepts presents any intellectual difficulty.

Learning is easier when interconnections between subjects are known. Within ophthalmology these are explained; for example, the association between refractive errors and other eye diseases. Even more important, the associations between ophthalmology and general medicine, especially neurology, are emphasized.

Interest is another important basis for learning and we hope that we give the impression that ophthalmology is fascinating, from optics to surgery, and from neuro-ophthalmology to epidemiology. The rate of advance in many areas of our subject, as in medicine, science and biology in general, has been so fast in recent years that subspecialization within it is increasing. Accordingly, even in a basic clinical text, several chapters have been contributed by authors on their own special interests; the first five chapters are interrelated, however, each building on information in previous ones, so they have been written by the editor. Some duplication between chapters has been permitted to allow continuity and reasonable completeness within chapters. It is a great pity that most medical students are given little opportunity for a study in depth, because of pressure of time: a few references are given to encourage them to go to the library of the department of ophthalmology where they will find a profusion of journals in many languages and a quickly accumulating collection of textbooks and monographs on broad and narrow aspects of the subject.

Ophthalmology is a colourful subject. We are grateful to Merck Sharp and Dohme for generous financial support towards the cost of the illustrations which will help the student in the diagnostic process much more than will pages of printed words.

One of our underlying objectives should be overtly stated: prevention of blindness. By spreading knowledge of our subject we hope that early diagnosis and rational management will contribute to a reduction in morbidity. However, we must always keep in mind the enormous difference between the relatively less important *unilateral* poor vision or blindness and the tragedy of *bilateral* blindness.

Teaching is a great art, and success can be achieved in various ways. A short introductory chapter, following this preface, presents some ideas which have been evolved over many years for undergraduate teaching, and we hope they will be useful for the junior clinician who often is also a clinical lecturer.

The last word which every clinical teacher would leave with his students is that the best way to learn a clinical subject is to sit down with the patient and take and record a careful, sympathetic history (not necessarily long), perform a selective unhurried examination, advise treatment with due regard to the risks involved, then keep the results under review, with an open mind on the validity of the original diagnosis and on the benefits of the treatment. Accordingly the best place to learn a clinical subject is the outpatient department, and we hope that this text will make the student's and teacher's and patient's task easier.

Contributors

John D C Anderson, OBE, MD, FRCS
Senior Lecturer, Department of Preventive Ophthalmology, Institute of Ophthalmology, University of London

Desmond B Archer, MD, FRCS
Professor of Ophthalmology, Queen's University, Belfast; Honorary Consultant Ophthalmic Surgeon, Royal Victoria Hospital, Belfast

Richard Collin, MA MB (Cantab), FRCS, DO
Consultant Surgeon, Moorfields Eye Hospital, London; Honorary Consultant Surgeon, Hospital for Sick Children, Great Ormond Street, London

Alexander L Crombie, MB (Ed), FRCS (Ed)
Professor of Ophthalmology and Associate Dean of the Medical School, University of Newcastle upon Tyne; Consultant Ophthalmologist, Royal Victoria Infirmary, Newcastle upon Tyne

Sidney Davidson, MB (Glas), FRCS, DO
Director of Studies, Department of Ophthalmology, University of Liverpool; Consultant Ophthalmic Surgeon, St Paul's Eye Hospital, Liverpool

David L Easty, MD, FRCS, DO
Professor of Ophthalmology, University of Bristol; Honorary Consultant Surgeon, Bristol Eye Hospital

Andrew R Elkington, MA (Cantab), MB, FRCS, DO
Consultant Surgeon, Southampton Eye Hospital; Senior Lecturer in Ophthalmology, University of Southampton

Paul Hunter, MA, MB (Cantab), FRCS, DO
Consultant Ophthalmic Surgeon, Kings College Hospital, London

Malcolm G Kerr-Muir, MB, MRCP, FRCS, DTM & H
Lecturer, Department of Clinical Ophthalmology, Moorfields Eye
Hospital, London

Calbert I Phillips, MD (Aberd), PHD (Bristol), MSC (Manc), DPH (Ed),
FRCS (Ed and Eng), DO, FBOA (Hon)
Professor of Ophthalmology, University of Edinburgh; Honorary
Consultant Ophthalmic Surgeon, Royal Infirmary, Edinburgh

Ian G Rennie, MB (Sheff), FRCS (Ed)
Lecturer in Ophthalmology, Department of Ophthalmology, University
of Liverpool; Honorary Senior Registrar, St Paul's Eye Hospital,
Liverpool

A G Tyers, MB (Lond), FRCS, FRCS (Ed), DO
Senior Registrar, Moorfields Eye Hospital, London

Acknowledgements

I am very grateful to Mr I Lennox, Department of Medical Illustration, University of Edinburgh, and Mr T R Tarrant of Moorfields Eye Hospital for their skill and patience in making the diagrams and paintings, and to Merck Sharp and Dohme for generously meeting the cost of the coloured illustrations. Miss Marion McCutcheon, my secretary, has been a very efficient and tolerant typist and organizer of the many revisions of the text.

General Suggestions for Teachers

(See the beginning of Chapters 2, 3 and 4 for more specific information)

The organization of the teaching of clinical ophthalmology for medical undergraduates, general practitioners, opticians, orthoptists and nurses will depend to some extent on the arrangements which have evolved in different universities, hospitals and training schools. The suggestions in this section can be modified to meet individual circumstances. They are based mainly on my teaching experience in the University of Manchester and, subsequently, in the University of Edinburgh. We are fortunate in Edinburgh to have small groups of undergraduate medical students (8–10 students in each group) allotted to our 80-bed hospital for a period of two weeks, but with no preceding lecture course. Within the first four half-days we present the contents of the first four chapters of this book, with tutorial and discussion. Presbyopia is an important part of Chapter 2, 'Clinical Examination of the Eye and Adnexa', which prepares the way for the explanation of hypermetropia in Chapter 3, which in turn is necessary to understand the mechanism of (accommodative) strabismus. The student can then add myopia, contrasting it with hypermetropia, in Chapter 4 and can then superimpose astigmatism, regular and irregular, on the other ametropias. Angle-closure glaucoma (Chapter 5) is easier to understand if the concept of hypermetropia is already clear. The order of the later subjects is less important.

During the two-week attachment, we circulate each student round all major hospital departments—general clinics, glaucoma and children's clinics, accident and emergency, artificial eye and orthoptic departments, ward rounds and the operation theatre. By far the most important of these is the general outpatient department where he spends four or five half-days, one student being with one clinician.

It is valuable for a student to be with an experienced clinician at work. During a clinic a student should take a history from, examine and diagnose at least two patients, recording all of this; allow him only 15–20 minutes per patient. Look at his written records and encourage clear writing and the recording of information about right and left eyes on separate halves of the page, so important throughout medicine (especially in orthopaedics!). Many will omit visual acuity, or will not make that the first part of the examination. The value of the pin-hole test can be emphasized on these occasions. It is very useful practically for each clinician's consulting room to have a second, simpler, set-up in the same room for testing visual acuity and examining the patient—if the room is large enough. Other interesting patients can be 'demonstrated' to the students during the clinic—if necessary interrupting his more detailed examination of his 'long' cases.

The patient's general health should always be considered in the ophthalmic assessment. Even if there is no (known) connection with the eye symptoms, his general health is important in the management of his eye disease; for example, his expectation of life in relation to a decision to operate on his cataracts. If you ask a student about the possible complications of cataract extraction, he will usually forget about systemic complications such as deep femoral vein occlusion and atelectasis and bronchopneumonia. Ophthalmology is also valuable to reinforce general medical teaching; for example, cardiovascular diseases, neurology, genetics, paediatrics and so on. Pharmacology is another very important common ground; for example, ophthalmic complications of steroids and chloroquine on the one hand, and, on the other hand, the systemic complications of topical eye treatment such as beta-blockers, atropine, etc.

The teaching of some ophthalmic pathology will help to ensure that ophthalmology is not regarded as different from the clinical sciences in general. A series of histology slides and microscopes and some pathological specimens, all with explanatory notes, provides a good opportunity for self-teaching.

Ophthalmic optics is rather different from other medical subjects and we are dependent on the student's memory of simple physics. Blackboard diagrams, like those in Chapters 2, 3 and 4, are easily understood. A demonstration of different sorts of spectacles is an important practical way of helping the student to 'diagnose' his patients' refractive errors— and the diseases with which they are associated.

To indicate the fascinating range and depth of the subject, and its speed of advance, a small collection of recently published books, journals or reprints in the seminar room is useful. These should be kept up to date. The annual report of the Medical Defence Union is a useful teaching vehicle!

To encourage a study in depth, and to help to break down the barriers between subjects, each student may be given a topic for a 1000 word essay to write during his two-week attachment. For example: 'Discuss chlamydial diseases', 'Discuss diagnosis and management of a girl of 20 who has just recovered from unilateral retrobulbar neuritis', 'Discuss the problem of genetic counselling for a man of 25 (adopted as a child) showing signs of retinitis pigmentosa'. To provide the student with an opportunity to practise 'giving a paper' and to 'think on his feet', the essay subject can be used for a five-minute presentation to the group at the end of the course. An alternative is to give a student a journal reference on a recent advance, general or ophthalmological, of which an abstract will be presented to the class. A better performance will be obtained if this occasion is part of the assessment, and a better discussion will be evoked if the audience are warned that their participation will be included as part of *their* assessment! The average British medical student tends to be too passive, a reflection on our teaching methods.

Examinations are a useful vehicle for teaching, as the above paragraph implies. A written paper lasting an hour can sample half a dozen parts of the subject: 'Write a short account of' stimulates the essay-writing centres which are tending to atrophy nowadays. A multiple choice questions (MCQ) paper can deal more easily with large numbers, and reduce the labour and subjectivity of marking.

Most important of all is a clinical examination, in which the student writes down a history from an actual patient, records his findings and writes down a diagnosis. Marks are allotted for recording of the findings as well as, of course, the quality of the history taking and clinical examination and accuracy of the clinical findings, diagnosis and management. There are two objectives in this clinical examination: one is to impress on the student's mind a particular patient; the other is to ensure that the student will attend the clinical sessions and apply himself during them. The student needs constant encouragement to involve himself with the patient.

Finally, the high quality of the teaching should inspire a few able students with steady hands, nimble fingers and full stereoscopic vision to spend a lifetime in an absorbing and varied subject with research potential in every part of it.

C I Phillips

1

Embryology, Anatomy and Physiology
An introduction

C I Phillips

The eyeballs are developed in early intrauterine life as outpouchings of a single cell layer from the forebrain vesicle, one on each side (*see* Plate 1.1). Their extremity lies under the surface ectoderm. These hollow 'optic vesicles' become indented ventrally, making the dorsal edge prominent. The primitive blood vessels on the surface of the optic vesicles, analogous to the superficial cortical vessels of the brain, remain on the inner concave surface of the indentation. Gradually the indentation deepens until a two-layer 'optic cup' is formed (*see* Plate 1.2). The indentation is called the fetal or ocular or choroidal cleft.

A defect in its closure, often inherited in a dominant pattern, produces a coloboma. Its most severe form consists of a wide area of missing retina and choroid extending from the optic disc, downwards of course, to the peripheral fundus: the ophthalmoscopist sees a large white area of 'bare' sclera involving most of the lower half of the fundus on both sides. The patient has bad vision and the eyes may be very small (microphthalmos). A segment of lower iris may be missing, alone or with a coloboma of fundus, but the whole pupil is also displaced downwards. There may be a notch at 6 o'clock in the lens. A mild form may be a white patch of two to three disc diameters inferiorly below the optic disc, often quite peripherally; similar patches in a right *and* left eye will support the diagnosis of a congenital partial coloboma. A common very minor form is represented by a small arc or crescent of missing choroid and retina just below the disc: survey your fellow students' fundi with an ophthalmoscope to establish its frequency. Another subclinical manifestation quite often visible in normal individuals is a darker patch of iris around 6 o'clock, usually bilaterally symmetrical.

The crystalline lens of the eye comes to lie in the mouth of the optic cup, having developed from a closed circle of ectodermal surface cells.

The related area of surface ectoderm develops into cornea and remains transparent throughout life (*see* Plate 1.3).

The deeper layer of the optic cup (now 'outer' from the point of view of the formed retina and eyeball) remains single-celled to become the pigment epithelium and Bruch's membrane of the retina. The inner layer, rather like the cerebral cortex to which it is analogous, develops into the retina proper with three main strata of cells. It is a quite extraordinary fact that it is the *outermost* stratum of this inner layer, next to the pigment epithelium, which is the light-sensitive one; it consists of rods and cones. Accordingly the innermost strata have to remain transparent!

Adult retina (Fig. 1.1)

A similarly odd arrangement places the retinal blood vessels on the inner surface of the retina where they interfere with the incident light—with remarkably little effect on visual function. Even the nuclei of the rod and cone cells lie on the *inner* side of their light-sensitive elements; that is, in

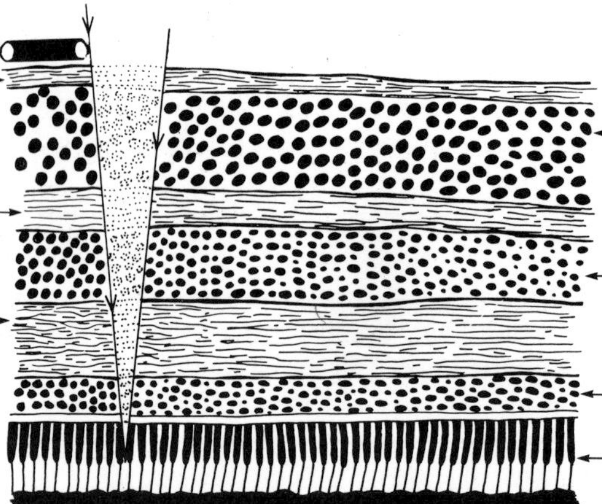

Fig 1.1 Diagram of a cross-section of retina, showing a clear wedge, base up, representing rays of light coming to a focus on the layer of rods which is almost the *deepest* layer of the retina—only the pigment epithelium and Bruch's membrane lie beyond it.

Note that the wedge of rays has just missed a retinal blood vessel as the wedge strikes the first layer of the retina constituted by axons of the ganglion cells as they pass towards the optic disc. The other layers contain mainly the following: 2. Ganglion cell layer; 3. Axons of cells in layers (2) and (4) both of which have synapses in this inner plexiform layer; 4. Bipolar cell layer—'inner nuclear layer'; 5. Axons of cells in layers (4) and (6), both of which have synapses in this 'outer plexiform layer'; 6. Cell bodies of the rods and cones—'outer nuclear layer'; 7. External limiting membrane—like wire netting with holes for the processes of the rods and cones; 8. Layer of rods and cones; 9. Retinal pigment epithelium.

the pathway of rays of light moving towards the outer segments of the rods and cones. A bipolar cell layer interposes itself between, and connects, on the outer side the rod and cone cell layer, and on the inner side the ganglion cell layer. The last forms a layer next to the cavity of the eyeball, which is filled up by transparent vitreous body (see Plate 1.4). The axons from the ganglion cells congregate at the optic nerve head (i.e. the optic disc) to escape from the eyeball through a perforated disc of sclera, after which they form the optic nerve in the orbit.

From the handicap of the 'back-to-front' arrangement of the retina— i.e. the placing of the light-sensitive cells (rods and cones) deeply, next to the pigment epithelium—Nature has extricated the retina with remarkable efficiency. The transparency of the layers of retina through which light rays have to pass has been achieved reasonably well throughout most of the retina, because resolution of the images need not be very detailed. The output from many (peripheral) rods contributes to one single ganglion cell, thereby minimizing the number of axons in the optic nerve and the amount of information to be processed by the brain. However, the macular area, with the *fovea centralis* at its centre, has a very high concentration of cones, and these have a one-to-one relationship with their ganglion cells (Fig 1.2). The macula is directly opposite the pupil and is designed to see detail in the centre of the field of vision. Accordingly, to continue the teleological* basis of the explanation, Nature has moved the bipolar and ganglion cell layer away from the fovea to allow more direct access of rays of light to the foveal cones; the corresponding bipolar and ganglion cells are 'heaped up' around the fovea.

The rods, mainly in the retinal periphery, respond to much lower levels of illumination than do the cones, which are concentrated in the macular area.

Uveal tract (see Plate 1.4)

This continuous layer of tissue, consisting of iris, ciliary body and choroid, is quite heavily pigmented with melanin (to exclude all rays of light from the eye except those entering via the pupil). The iris is highly 'elastic' and has a sphincter muscle surrounding the pupil (parasympathetic) and a dilator muscle (sympathetic). The ciliary body consists of a mass of ciliary muscle important in accommodation (Chapter 2) and a ciliary epithelium covering finger-like process, which increase its surface area, important in glaucoma (Chapter 5). The choroid

* Teleological means 'implying a design or purpose'.

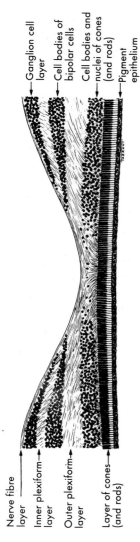

Nerve fibre layer

Inner plexiform layer

Outer plexiform layer

Layer of cones (and rods)

Ganglion cell layer

Cell bodies of bipolar cells

Cell bodies and nuclei of cones (and rods)

Pigment epithelium

Fig 1.2 Diagram of cross-section of retina at the fovea centralis of the macula. Nature has 'shifted' all possible nuclei and axons away from the fovea centralis, hence its concave inner surface. Accordingly, interference with rays of light being focused on this high-resolution area is minimized.

is very vascular, and leaky, and is responsible for exchanges with the metabolically highly active outer layer of the retina, the rods and cones.

Retrolental fibroplasia is an iatrogenic disease of babies, relevant here. Until late in intrauterine life, the thin retina can obtain all its nutrition from the choroid so that no separate retinal circulation needs to develop. When the retina thickens in the late months of pregnancy, oxygen from the choroid is no longer sufficient and retinal blood vessels grow from the optic disc to supply the inner layers of retina. If a child is born prematurely and is given a high concentration of oxygen to breathe, the choroidal blood vessels can supply more of the retina than usual so that the stimulus to development of the retinal circulation disappears and that separate system of blood vessels atrophies. When the child is removed from oxygen, the choroidal oxygen supply is suddenly inadequate and there is marked retinal anoxia, to which the blood vessels from the disc respond with vigorous unorganized proliferation—into retina and vitreous—along with fibrous tissue. Contraction of fibrous tissue in retina and vitreous can quickly cause total retinal detachment and permanent blindness. Milder cases can occur.

Further details of anatomy and physiology will be found in the chapters on special subjects.

2

Clinical Examination of the Eye and Adnexa

C I Phillips

Suggestions for teachers

As the students assemble for the first tutorial, instil tropicamide (Mydriacyl) 1% into one eye, right or left at random, having warned them through the dean's office previously not to drive cars that day. Demonstrate and explain the technique of instillation, emphasizing precautions against cross-infection. Towards the end of the first tutorial, their pupils will be dilated and enough paralysis of accommodation obtained so that you will be able to teach the students on themselves:

1   *about presbyopia and its correction;*
2   *something about mydriatics and cycloplegics and drug penetration into the eye;*
3   *(a) how to use focal illumination — e.g. to see the cornea, anterior chamber and the anterior and posterior surfaces of the lens and its thickness,*
    (b) how to do direct ophthalmoscopy which is so much easier on the eye with the dilated pupil.

Essential equipment is one ophthalmoscope for each pair of students: suppliers seem happy to lend instruments. One +3 dioptre lens per pair of students demonstrates the impressive treatment of the 'presbyopia' induced by tropicamide. Consider in advance how you will teach ophthalmoscopy to one-eyed students (see below). Slit-lamp microscopy is excluded here, but a student in the outpatient or accident and emergency department will be interested to use it occasionally — the extra-viewer attachment for the Haag–Streit slit-lamp saves the clinician much time.

History taking

History taking is the most important part of any clinical assessment in any subject. Experience, with knowledge, will help in learning the art of eliciting the important points, and the art of saving time by only brief enquiry about other areas. The reader should extract from each part of this book the presenting symptoms of every disease, and this will allow him to direct his attention in the examination to particular parts of the eye and surrounding structures. The importance of the general health must be emphasized: even if it is of little *direct* relevance, at the very least it is important in decisions about management of the eye disease — e.g. expectation of life in cases of cataract or glaucoma. The testing of visual acuity and ophthalmoscopy are two examinations which the ophthalmologist does on every patient. Others, such as ocular movements, cover test, pupil reactions and testing of fields of vision are done only when the history indicates the need, and will be described in the appropriate chapters.

The student should try to take histories from, and examine, as many patients as possible. By that means he will quickly become an experienced clinician who starts the diagnostic process during the history by pattern recognition — i.e. by applying Bayes's theorem*.

Then follows a selective clinical examination to refute or confirm the probable diagnosis, or diagnoses in their order of preference — an application of one of Karl Popper's† principles [1]. Diagnostic logic is not a difficult or complicated process. There should be minimal dependence on laboratory tests, x-rays and other special investigations: their results are often of little discriminatory value (and are often equivocal), sometimes positively deleterious or hazardous, and always expensive.

Visual acuity

The visual acuity must be recorded in each eye separately in all patients who have visual symptoms, and should be recorded in others as part of a

---

* The basic form of the theorem of the Rev Thomas Bayes (1701–1760), applied to diagnostic logic is:

$$P(D/S) = \frac{P(S/D) \times P(D)}{P(S)}$$

This formula says that the probability (P) of a diagnosis or disease (D) *given* (vertical bar) the symptoms and signs (S) is equal to the probability of the symptoms and signs *given* the diagnosis multiplied by the probability of the diagnosis (i.e. the frequency in the parent population) divided by the probability of the symptoms and signs (i.e. the frequency of symptoms and signs whether or not the disease exists). The term $P(D)$ is the 'prior probability' (e.g. very small for a diagnosis of malaria in Western Europe but very high in some countries). (*See* Lindley D (1971) *Making Decisions.* New York and Chichester: Interscience).

† Karl Popper (b. 1902): Emeritus Professor of Logic and Scientific Method, University of London.

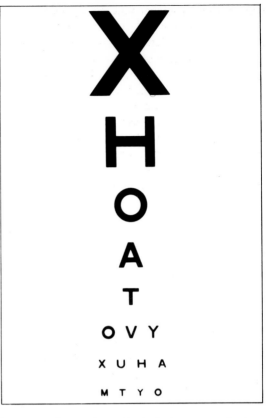

Fig 2.1 Snellen's test chart. The top letter can be seen by a normal eye at 60 metres, the next at 36 metres, next 24 metres, then 18, 12, 9 (there are three letters in that row), 6, 5 metres. 'VAR 6/18 without spectacles' means that at a distance of 6 metres from the chart, the patient's right eye, uncorrected optically, can only manage to see a line the normal eye can see at 18 metres. This chart can be used with a mirror if a room with only a 3 metres dimension is available, since the letters are symmetrical about a vertical axis. The use of single letters down to and including the 12 metre line saves the examiner much time.

thorough general medical examination. It is particularly important in the diagnosis of cataract in the elderly, the usual presenting symptom being blurred vision. It is essential in the assessment of squint in the young. A normal visual acuity implies a clear lens, and also clear cornea and vitreous, and a normally functioning macular area of the retina along with intact neural pathways to and in the brain leading to the occipital cortex and beyond to the higher centres concerned with interpretation of patterns. It gives little information about fields of vision.

Snellen's test chart

A Snellen's test chart is placed on a wall 6 metres in front of the patient (Fig. 2.1). If only a shorter distance is available, a mirror is sited 3 metres in front of the patient so that he can see a chart with 'reversed' letters placed above his head (or a chart with letters symmetrical about a vertical axis, e.g. X but not E). The image of the test chart is effectively 3 metres behind the mirror; that 3 metres is added to the 3 metres' distance between the patient and the mirror so that the standard 6 metres is obtained. The top letter is so big that it could be seen by a normal eye at a distance of 60 metres (USA, 200 feet!), the next line at a distance of 36 metres, the next at 24, next at 18, then 12, 9, 6, 5 and even on some charts 4 metres. A patient who has normal visual acuity and is sited 6 metres from the chart will see the '6 metre line', and often the 5 or 4 metre line.

Always start the eye examination with the visual acuity. *Always test the right eye first*, then the left, because when you go to write down your findings you will remember the result from the *first* eye tested and that from the *second* eye but not which side until you are more experienced. First, cover the left eye with a card or diary, tilted to ensure that there is no possibility that the covered left eye can see the chart. This is sometimes difficult in children. Ask the patient to read out the letters from the top: the last complete line he reads indicates the visual acuity (VA). Then test the left eye and record the results thus:

VAR 6/18 with spectacles   VAL 6/5 with spectacles

The '6' indicates the patient's distance in metres from the test chart, and the other figure the distance at which a normal eye can see the lowest line the patient can see; 6/6 (USA 20/20; i.e. in feet) is the minimum normal standard. Always specify with or without *distance* spectacles and, if the patient has distance spectacles, do not bother to test his VA without spectacles. Note that *any* information about the *right* eye is recorded on the *left* side of the page, as in other specialties—as if the patient is looking at you out of the page. This is a most important aid to preventing a mix-up between right and left eyes, which can be disastrous.

Many patients have a VA of less than 6/60 yet are not 'blind' in the clinical sense, especially if they have intact peripheral fields. In practice, the ophthalmologist rarely moves the patient gradually metre by metre nearer to the chart till he can see the top letter—VA being 5/60, 4/60, 3/60, 2/60 or 1/60 respectively. He prefers to ask the patient if he can count the number of his fingers spread at 1 metre or 0.5 metre (VA = CF at 1 m or 0.5 m). The next lower stage is 'hand movements' (HM) at 1 metre or 0.5 metre or 0.25 metre; then 'perception of light' (PL) if the patient can tell the examiner when a torchlight is shone into the pupil (note whether the pupil constricts to light) and then turned away. Finally 'no perception of light' (no PL) may be the acuity which has to be recorded; this is 'blind' in the clinical and pathological senses (but see Chapter 17 for definition of 'blindness' for the UK social services).

A pin-hole test will improve the patient's visual acuity by several lines on the chart if his poor performance is due to a refractive error; other conditions will allow no improvement. The explanation is that a pin-hole in a disc (easily available in all boxes of trial lenses, or easily contrived by perforating a card with a thick pin), held as close as possible to the eye, eliminates the effect of the eye's lens system. (A pin-hole camera can produce an image without a lens.)

Even if a patient's visual acuity is only PL, it is important to test whether there is good 'projection of light—i.e. to test the fields of vision. As the patient looks straight ahead in a semi-dark room, shine a moderately bright beam of light obliquely into his pupil randomly from four different directions (his upper left, lower left, upper right and lower right) and ask him to 'point to where my light is coming from' with his forefinger.

Fields of vision

These are being tested as described above when the patient has poor acuity. When visual acuity is good, it is often useful to test the fields quickly to finger movements, to exclude large defects in his fields of vision. Ask the patient to cover his left eye, holding the upper lid down with his left fingers. Tell him to look with his right eye at the point of your (the examiner's) nose. In the middle of each quadrant of his right field at random (upper right, lower right, upper left, lower left) flutter your index and middle fingers (noiselessly!) and ask him to 'point to the fingers that are moving'. Then test his left eye.

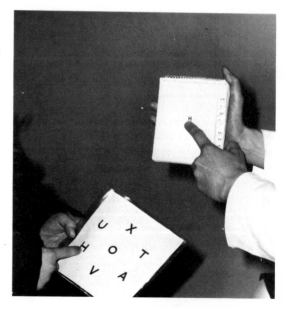

Fig 2.2 Sheridan–Gardiner test. Actual distance between patient and test card should be 6 metres. A preschool child can recognize shapes of X, O, H etc. without knowing them as letters, hence this is a useful test of visual acuity for young children.

Illiterates

Illiterates form a high proportion of the population: almost all children under the age of 6 years. But patients with dyslexia or nominal aphasia are rare. A Sheridan–Gardiner test is commonly used for children (Fig 2.2). The examiner stands 6 metres away and shows one easily recognized pattern at a time (e.g. H or X) and the child is merely required to point to the same shape out of a small group of letters printed on a card in his own or his mother's hand; he is *not* expected to say what letter it is, and children of 2½ or 3 years can usually co-operate easily. Other methods are used for younger children.

Near vision and presbyopia

When Snellen's test chart is used for *distance* vision, rays of light from the chart are very nearly parallel as they enter the pupil of the eye, 6 metres being infinity for practical purposes. The normal eye is constructed so that, with accommodation entirely relaxed, these rays will be brought to a focus on the retina by the very high refractive power of the cornea, which is around 43 dioptres, and the lesser power of the crystalline lens within the eye, which is around 17 dioptres. (The power of a lens in dioptres is the reciprocal of the focal length expressed in metres.) In contrast, at the usual reading distance of about 0.33 metre, rays of light from a near object are diverging as they enter the pupil (Fig 2.3). To avoid

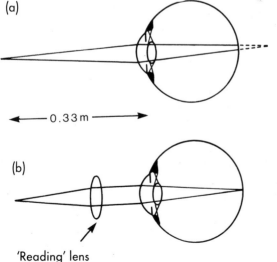

(a)

← 0.33 m →

(b)

'Reading' lens

Fig 2.3 Presbyopia.
(a) Rays of light are diverging quite strongly from an object—e.g. the letters on the page of a book situated 0.33 metre in front of the eye. In white patients over 45 years (in many races over 35), the ciliary muscle cannot alter the shape of the lens sufficiently from oval towards round (to make the curvatures of the surface steeper) to bring these rays of light to a focus on the retina.
(b) A positive (biconvex) spectacle lens is required for reading.

a blurred image of a near object on the retina, the ciliary muscle contracts so that the suspensory ligament of the lens is slackened off, and the lens indulges its natural tendency to get fatter (= accommodation). Its surface curvatures become steeper, and angulate the rays of light more as they pass through. Provided that 3 dioptres of accommodation (1/0.33 m) are available, the eye will produce a clear image on the retina of an object 0.33 metre from it.

At the age of 8 years the power of accommodation is around 14 dioptres, giving a near point of (1/14 × 100) cm = 7.1 cm. The ability of the lens to change its shape gradually diminishes throughout life because of an increase in the density of packing of the cells in the lens itself, along with loss of elastic recoil in the capsule: the ciliary muscle cannot overcome these changes in spite of an increase in muscular effort. *Around 45 years in caucasians and often 35 in others, the near point has receded to 0.33 metre and so the symptom of blurred print (while wearing distance glasses if any) appears in practically 100% of the population.* At this stage 'presbyopia' ('old age vision'!) has started. Accommodation continues to diminish progressively until the age of around 65 years when none usually remains.

Accordingly, reading spectacles have to be used (Fig 2.4). At 65 years and over, a +3 dioptre lens is then theoretically required to see print etc.

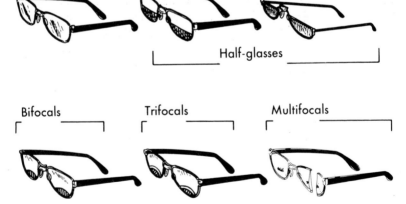

Fig 2.4 Available forms of lenses for treatment of presbyopia. Top left shows ordinary reading spectacles which have to be taken off when clear distance vision is required. Half-glasses allow the emmetrope to see distant objects clearly over the tops of the reading lenses. Bifocals allow the ametrope to see clearly for distance and, when looking downwards, for near. Bifocals can be supplied with clear glass for distance. Trifocals give the advanced presbyope clear vision at three different distances. With multifocals, the advanced presbyope can see clearly at any distance by tilting his head or moving his direction of gaze. Multifocal lenses are ground to have a *gradually* increasing dioptric power from the intercept of the visual axes with the lens for a distant object downwards to the intercept for reading.

clearly at 0.33 metre, but most patients are comfortable with a +2.75D lens or a +2.75D arithmetic addition to distance spectacles. At 45 years, only a +0.75D power is required. It is clinically and economically good practice to see the patient around age 52 to prescribe a +1.5D lens approximately and around 58, say, for a +2.25D lens and finally, at 65 years for a +2.75D lens—and to check the optic discs for pathological cupping.

To put on and take off reading glasses frequently is awkward, so that bifocals often, trifocals rarely, or multifocals sometimes, are used (Fig 2.4). The 'distance' part of the lens may be plain glass (i.e. for an emmetrope).

Near vision should be tested on near vision test types with reading spectacles if worn. The smallest print is labelled N5 and corresponds to the smallest size of newspaper print—which can be substituted if no proper test type is available. As in the case of Snellen's test type, increasing sizes of print are used to measure precisely this important function.

Ophthalmoscopy

An ophthalmoscope is a torch with a narrow bright beam, designed to allow the user to look along the centre of the beam and to see an illuminated area. So that the illuminated area can be in focus for the observer, a changeable series of lenses is incorporated on a rotating disc to compensate for refractive errors in the patient's or observer's eye.

The two most important uses of the ophthalmoscope are:

1   to detect opacities in the normally transparent media of the eye—i.e. in the cornea, crystalline lens and vitreous;
2   to examine the fundus of the eye, especially retina and optic disc (optic nerve head).

Pupil-dilating (mydriatic) and ciliary muscle-paralysing (cycloplegic) drugs for ophthalmoscopy

The fundus of the eye, especially the macular area, is much easier to examine if the pupil is dilated. To minimize inconvenience, a quick-action short-duration but powerful mydriatic is best. Tropicamide 1% or 0.5% has moderate anticholinergic activity and so weakens the sphincter pupillae and the ciliary muscle: the tone of the dilator muscle of the iris is enough then to produce mydriasis, but active stimulation of it by phenylephrine 10%, a sympathomimetic, will be supplementary. The main effect of both drugs will have passed off in 4–6 hours, during which time the patient should be advised to avoid car-driving. Other anticholinergic drugs are cyclopentolate (Mydrilate) 1% and homatropine 1% whose effects last for 24 hours; unfortunately; atropine's effect lasts for several days.

One small risk exists in producing mydriasis, and that is in eyes predisposed to angle-closure glaucoma (*see* Chapter 5). An acute attack of angle-closure glaucoma may be produced: indeed a mydriatic provocative test is sometimes used in its diagnosis. These eyes are small, and have shallow anterior chambers and small diameter corneas: ask if any first degree relatives required an emergency eye operation. If in doubt, avoid a mydriatic, or dilate one pupil only at one visit and ensure that the pupil has been re-constricted by guttae pilocarpine 0.5% or 1% before the patient leaves.

To detect opacities in the media (Right eye; Fig 2.5)

Stand on the patient's right and hold your ophthalmoscope in your right hand. Put a zero lens in the peep-hole if you are emmetropic, or wear your distance spectacles, or put your own spectacle correction in the peep-hole if you prefer to take off your spectacles. Place your *left* hand

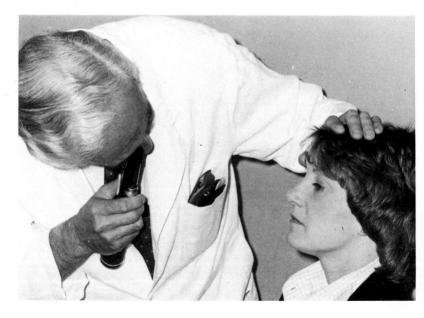

Fig 2.5 Detecting opacities in media with ophthalmoscope. See text.

on the patient's head so that your left thumb can lift his right upper lid. Position the ophthalmoscope close to your right eye so that you can look through the peep-hole along the beam of light. Imagine that the head of the ophthalmoscope is welded to your face—movement between the two should be almost completely avoided, although movements of your head plus ophthalmoscope as a single entity are very important. From a distance of about 0.5 metre (i.e. about half an arm's length) shine the light into the patient's pupil and note the even yellowish-red 'reflex' which fills the pupil—a reflection of the reddish colour from the fundus.

Any central corneal or lens or vitreous opacity will show up as a black silhouette on the yellow-red background (see Plate 8.1). Even slight abnormalities will be revealed in this way: for example, some corneal opacities which cannot easily be seen by 'focal' illumination (see below). The position of such an opacity relative to the pupil, and its apparent movement with change in the observer's viewpoint, will indicate the plane of the opacity—e.g. cornea or vitreous (Fig 2.6). If the observer moves his head plus ophthalmoscope as a unit, but maintains the light directed into the pupil, an opacity in the anterior lens capsule (i.e. in the plane of the pupil) will show no apparent movement in relation to the pupil margins. However, if the central opacity is in the posterior vitreous and, say, the observer moves his head upwards to look down from above, the central vitreous opacity will appear to move upwards towards the upper edge of the pupil and will quickly disappear behind it. The further from the plane of the pupil, the faster the apparent movement. If the

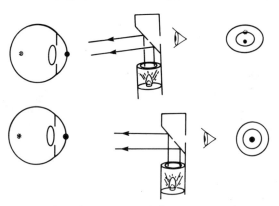

Fig 2.6 Parallactic displacement to estimate position of opacities in media. The lower diagram shows how an axial opacity at any depth will appear in the centre of the pupil to an observer directly in front of the patient's eye. In the upper diagram, if the observer plus ophthalmoscope moves upwards, a corneal opacity will appear to move slightly downwards and a posterior vitreous opacity will appear to move quickly upwards. No apparent movement will occur with an opacity in or near the plane of the pupil (e.g. a cataract in the lens) although a posterior lens opacity will appear to move slowly.

central opacity is in the cornea it will appear to move downwards—relatively slowly.

Do not be confused by an image of retinal vessels which can often be seen—they appear to move very fast of course—or minor vague areas of darkness, discs or doughnuts, which are due to variations in refractive index of the nucleus of lens etc. Pay attention to dense black silhouettes.

To examine the patient's *left* eye, stand on the patient's *left* and use your own *left* eye with the ophthalmoscope in your left hand; i.e. substitute left for right throughout the above description. If you are one-eyed, or have difficulty in shutting one eye, you will have to examine both the patient's eyes with your usable eye (*see* below). Most right-handed and right-eyed people need a little practice to master the use of their left eye.

Fundus examination

Close attention to three points will make this much easier:

1 space for the observer to move freely on each side of the patient;
2 stance;
3 the 'nose-on-knuckle' principle.

Right eye (Fig 2.7)
Sit the patient comfortably in a chair, looking straight ahead at some obvious target at about eye level; e.g. Angle-poise lamp, letters on the test chart, centre of a wall. Do not let the patient try to help by tilting his head back or turning it to right or left. Ensure that, for about 1 metre on each side of the patient, there is nothing to obstruct your free movement—or have the patient sit in a rotating chair to let you achieve free space on his right, then left.

You will usually prefer to remove your own spectacles unless you are significantly astigmatic and so you must modify the dioptres mentioned below by your spectacle correction. For example, if you are a −3D myopic, you will see the fundus clearly with a −3D lens in the peep-hole, not a zero lens.

Stand *on the patient's right* so that the patient's *right* eyeball is opposite your *left* heel (Fig 2.7). A line joining your right and left toes should be parallel to the patient's line of sight. Golfers will recognize the similarity of the stance for driving a ball from the tee. *Do not stand in front of the patient at all.*

Again, place your *left* hand flat on the patient's head and lift his right upper lid with your thumb, *bending the first knuckle of your thumb.*

Rotate the lens disc of your ophthalmoscope until a +12 or +10

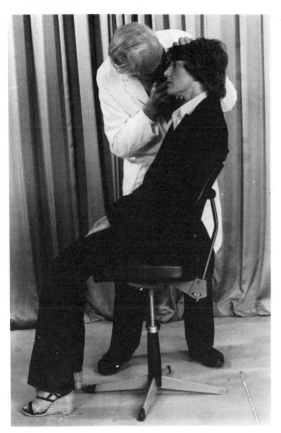

Fig 2.7 Stance for viewing the fundus with the ophthalmoscope. The observer uses his right eye for the patient's right eye (left for left). As for a tee shot with a driver, the patient's eyeball is opposite the examiner's left heel: a line joining the tips of his toes is parallel with the patient's visual axis.

dioptre lens is in the peep-hole and position the ophthalmoscope close to your right eye so that you can see through the peep-hole.

Approximate the ophthalmoscope plus observer's head as a single entity to the patient's right eye so that you can look through the patient's pupil — i.e. with the ophthalmoscope about 2.5 cm from the patient's eye (Fig 2.8). Nearer can be dangerous for the eye, and further away reduces your field of vision too much. The correct distance can usually be achieved by placing *the side of your nose on the bent knuckle of your thumb* and using that fixed point as a pivot for your wide-ranging examination of the fundus. That 'nose-on-knuckle' trick is *very* important. Because the observer's head and face are oblique to the patient's, the top of the observer's head will inevitably interfere with the patient's view of the target from his left eye. Accordingly, just before you look in through his pupil, tell the patient to 'look in the direction of the letters [or whatever target you have chosen] and keep looking in that

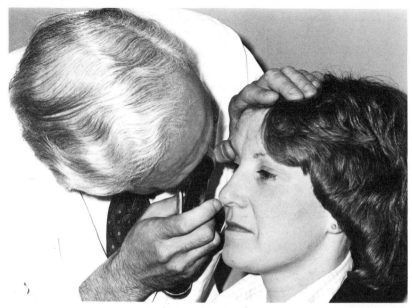

Fig 2.8 The observer achieves the correct distance for ophthalmoscopy by placing his nose on the bent knuckle of his thumb which is holding up the patient's upper lid.

direction even though my head gets in the way'. Very, very few patients find this difficult.

When you are in the correct position you will see a yellowish-red reflex from the fundus, blurred because of that +12D or +10D lens in the ophthalmoscope. With it, you can see in focus any opacity in the normally transparent cornea, or more often in the lens (i.e. cataract). Turn the disc of lenses of the ophthalmoscope through the range of lenses quite quickly, +10, +8, +7, +6 etc., thinking of the plane of anterior lens, posterior lens, anterior, middle and posterior vitreous respectively, and survey for any opacities in these planes. Move your head plus ophthalmoscope slightly as you focus deeper into the eye in order to impose apparent movement on any opacities, and so make them more easily seen.

Continue turning the disc of lenses (+4 etc.) *until you can just see clearly a blood vessel on the fundus.* For an emmetropic patient and observer, the 0 (zero) lens should be in the peep-hole: to 0 can be added arithmetically the patient's distance correction (say +2) and also the observer's (say −3) with a resultant −1D (0 + 2 − 3) in the peep-hole. The observer *can* continue to see the fundus clearly, even though he racks on to −2, −3, −4 etc. lenses, by exerting his own accommodation to compensate, but this is an uncomfortable process which is to be avoided.

Having identified a blood vessel clearly, you should follow it back a short way to its origin, at the optic disc—usually very easy to do, but occasionally difficult for the beginner. Provided that the patient is sitting as described, you will find that the optic disc will appear if you direct your gaze towards the left occipital pole or mastoid process.

Always examine the fundus systematically as follows, A, B, C and D:

A. Disc. When you have found the disc, consider its properties under the heading three Cs:

C for colour: pale or pink?
C for contour: are the edges sharp all round or blurred?
C for cupping: how big is the cup in relation to the disc—i.e. physiological or pathologically large?

B. Vessels. From the disc, follow the superotemporal, inferotemporal, superonasal and inferonasal vessels outwards from the disc, looking for calibre variations, white sheaths (rarely), both due to atherosclerosis, nearby haemorrhages and exudates. However, the easiest way to differentiate many retinopathies is to take the blood pressure and test the urine for sugar!

C. Fundus periphery should be quickly scanned as far out as possible. Ask the patient to look up to the ceiling; turn-tilt your head so that your

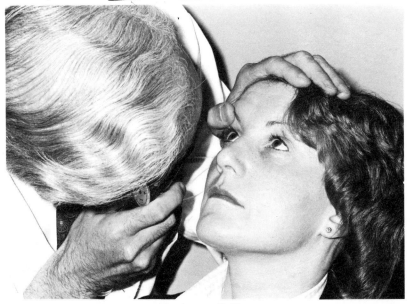

Fig 2.9 To see the upper fundus, the patient looks up and the observer tilts his occiput towards the floor.

occiput points towards the floor and so your direction of gaze is upwards to see the 12 o'clock area of the fundus (Fig 2.9). Then ask the patient to look downwards, then to right and to left, orientating your head and therefore your gaze appropriately, scanning the areas between these points as you change your direction of gaze.

D. *The macula* should be examined last because the patient is dazzled by the light (*see* Fig 1.2). You will find it 2.5 disc diameters on the temporal side of the optic disc; alternatively, just ask the patient to look directly 'into the middle of the light'. The macular area is free from blood vessels and is slightly more pigmented than other areas of the fundus. Its centre, the fovea centralis, is much thinner than other areas of the posterior pole, because the bipolar and ganglion cells are moved away from it (and heaped up around it) to allow unobstructed access of light to the cones which are in high concentration. The concavity so produced acts as a concave mirror for the ophthalmoscope's beam, which is concentrated to produce a bright spot of light just in front of the macula (Fig 2.10): note the parallax between the spot of light and the fundus if you move your head plus ophthalmoscope slightly.

Left eye
To examine the left eye, substitute left for right in all the above instructions.

If you cannot learn to see with your right and left eyes reasonably equally (but you should try hard), you will have to examine both eyes of the patient

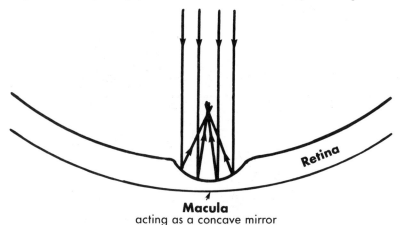

Macula
acting as a concave mirror

Fig 2.10 Some of the rays of light from the ophthalmoscope striking the retina in the macular area are reflected back as from a concave mirror to produce a bright yellow spot seen by the ophthalmoscopist (*see* Fig 1.2). If he moves his head plus ophthalmoscope, he will see, because of parallax, that the focused point of light is in front of the retina.

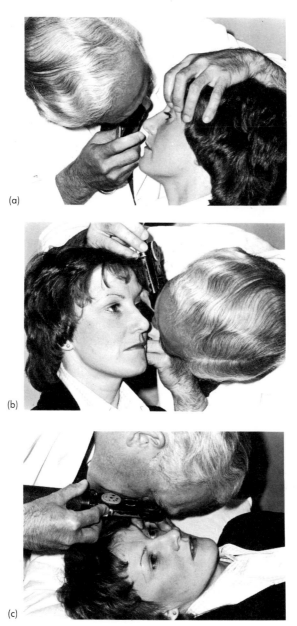

Fig 2.11 Ophthalmoscopist with poor left vision examining patient's left eye with his right in various ways: (a) leaning across while standing on patient's right;

(b) standing on patient's left; (c) patient lying on couch, observer standing behind her head (a low chair can be used).

with your usable eye. Suppose you cannot use your left eye. To examine the patient's left eye with your right, I recommend that you stand on the patient's right side, as for examining his right eye, but lean across his face with your forehead–chin axis at right angles to his, so that your noses do not clash. Your left eye will be directed to the middle of his left forehead (Fig 2.11a). Another way is to stand on his *left* side and again turn your forehead–chin axis at right angles to his—so that your left eye is looking at the middle of his cheek; the handle of your ophthalmoscope is directed skywards and you can rest your right hand on the patient's forehead (Fig 2.11b). Yet another way is to stand behind the patient seated on a low chair and lean over his head, your right eye to his left eye. Finally, the patient may be on a couch with you standing behind the top of the patient's head, facing the patient's feet: you then bend over the patient, your right eye to the patient's left (Fig 2.11c).

Focal illumination

A very bright focused light is obviously required to see details of the iris and cornea, conjunctiva and eyelid margins. The observer, using his reading spectacles if any, must bring his eye close to the patient's in order to obtain as much magnification as possible. A common fault is to fail to lift the upper lid which covers the upper cornea—and may hide a small corneal foreign body.

Most ophthalmoscopes provide for a focused light beam, but a pen-torch with a focusing bulb is almost as good. Note that through a dilated pupil, a fine focused beam can demonstrate the full thickness of the crystalline lens.

Reference

1 Campbell E J M (1976) Basic science, science and medical education. *Lancet* **1**, 134–6

3 Squint (Strabismus)

C I Phillips

Suggestions for teachers

It is useful to allot an individual student to an individual orthoptist for an hour or so, to see visual acuity being tested in children and to give him the opportunity to practise the cover/uncover test on patients, under supervision.

However, the orthoptist should not go into complicated details of orthoptic investigation and treatment. 'Fixation' by a squinting eye on the optic disc/blind spot might be explained. A Hess chart/Hess screen might be demonstrated. A receptive student might be interested in the mechanism of eccentric fixation.

The experimental basis of strabismic and deprivation amblyopias established by 1981 Nobel prizewinners Hubel and Wiesel is very relevant [1].

A useful working definition is that a squint exists when both visual axes do not intersect the point of visual attention. (For present purposes, the visual axis can be regarded as a line joining the object or fixation point, the centre of the pupil and the fovea centralis.) It is 'convergent' when one visual axis is turned medially (i.e. inwards, towards the nose) and 'divergent' if the visual axis is turned laterally (i.e. outwards). It is 'concomitant' if the abnormal angle between the visual axes remains approximately constant in all directions of gaze: this is the situation in the common squint in childhood. A good example of an 'incomitant' squint is a lateral rectus paralysis because the abnormal angle between the visual axes exists only in the direction towards which the paralysed muscle normally pulls the eye—for example, to the right in a right lateral rectus paralysis; in all other directions, both visual axes are directed successfully towards the object of attention.

Concomitant squint

Convergent

In the last chapter, mention was made of accommodation which results from contraction of the ciliary muscle within the eyeball. The suspensory ligament of the lens is slackened so that the lens becomes rounder (i.e. has more curved surfaces and therefore has a greater refractive power); accordingly, reading or close work become possible. An additional property of close work is important: convergence of the visual axes must occur to intersect at the point of attention (Fig 3.1).

In normal or emmetropic eyes, the exact amount of stimulus to convergence is sent down from the IIIrd nerve nucleus to correspond with the amount of accommodation exerted.

Now, hypermetropia is quite a common refractive error. In it, a relatively small eyeball has a lens system not strong enough to bring parallel rays of light to a focus on the retina (Fig 3.2). Such a pair of eyes will be able to see clearly for distance if some accommodation is exerted, but unfortunately convergence will also be stimulated. When these eyes look at a near object, the accommodation exerted will be greater than in the case of emmetropia, *and also convergence will be greater*. In many cases of hypermetropia this unstable situation, precariously maintained by binocular single vision, 'breaks down' into a convergent squint,

Fig 3.1 The medial recti are contracting (⟩⟨) to *converge the visual axes* by the correct amount for the amount of accommodation being exerted. 'Accommodation' (i.e. contraction of the ciliary muscle) is adding to the dioptric power of the lens the extra optical power required to *focus the rays* from a near object on the macula.

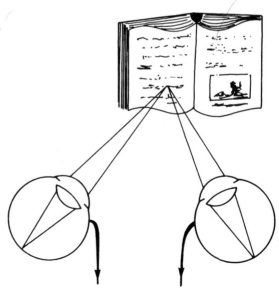

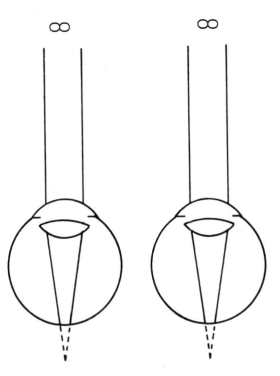

Fig 3.2 A pair of hypermetropic (long-sighted) eyes looking at an infinitely distant point (∞): parallel rays of light enter the pupils. Since accommodation is relaxed, a blurred image will be produced on both retinae. When accommodation is exerted to see clearly, convergence is also stimulated, even for distance, but especially for close work— with a risk of convergent squint.

especially if one eye is more hypermetropic or astigmatic than the other. There is some evidence that the amount of convergence per unit of accommodation is greater than usual in such cases. If the hypermetropia is equal in the two eyes, the right or left eye may squint indiscriminately—an 'alternating' squint. This explanation of the aetiological mechanism of the usual case of convergent strabismus is an oversimplification because many hypermetropes do not squint—and some emmetropes have a convergent squint.

A warning is appropriate here. Before deciding that a squint belongs to the 'concomitant' category, the examiner *must* exclude an 'incomitant' squint (*see* below)—e.g. due to a lateral rectus paralysis. Ocular movements should be carefully tested in all squints—the patient must watch an object (pen, torch, picture held in the examiner's hand) as it is moved right, left, up and down: it is usually wise to test each eye separately—i.e. cover one eye with your hand while you test the movements of the uncovered eye.

Occasionally a unilateral concomitant convergent squint *results* from bad vision in one eye in a child. If one eye has bad vision, binocular vision must be poor, with the result that a breakdown to overconvergence of that eye is likely. Possible causes are (congenital) cataract or unilateral corneal opacity or intrauterine toxoplasmic choroiditis at one macula or, rarely, a retinoblastoma in one eye. Because of these possibilities, the ophthalmologist *must* always examine both eyes carefully, especially the fundi, in all cases of squint *at the first visit*. In an adult, an eye which becomes blind usually *diverges*.

The immediate result of an accommodative squint is loss of binocular vision, the highest grade of which is stereoscopic vision (stereopsis). In a child, the transient diplopia which he presumably suffers is quickly eliminated by suppression of the area of retina responsible for the diplopic image and also suppression at the macular area of the squinting eye. Visual acuity deteriorates quickly. This important condition is called 'strabismic amblyopia', and the longer it is present and the younger the child affected, the more difficult it is to treat, and binocularity may also be permanently lost.

Occlusion (i.e. covering) of the normal eye by a patch actually stuck on the face will produce improvement in the visual acuity of the eye with strabismic amblyopia provided that the patient is under 6 or 7 years of age (Fig 3.3). The child may have the occlusion on the spectacle lens if he does not 'peep' round the side of the occluder. *Over the age of 6 or 7 years, improvement is very unlikely, and there is a definite danger of permanent diplopia.* In a child of 1 year with a recent squint, a week of occlusion may cure the amblyopia. In a child of 4 years with a squint of 2+ years' duration, improvement may take many weeks, and normal visual acuity may never be retrieved.

Fig 3.3 Occlusion on the face covers the normal right eye to stimulate the left to overcome its strabismic amblyopia.

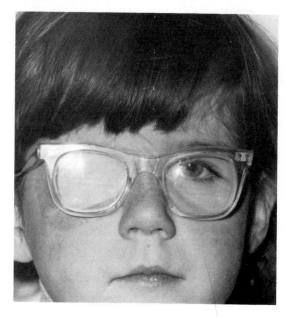

Operation for a convergent squint is one of the commonest eye operations. The insertion of the medial rectus to the eyeball is mobilized and it is reattached by two or three sutures to the sclera about 4–5 mm behind its normal insertion, to 'weaken' the muscle. In addition, a length of lateral rectus 5, 6, 7 or 8 mm long is often excised to 'strengthen' that muscle. In a squint of large angle, the fellow eye may require a similar operation. Some surgeons operate at a young age with the objective of retrieving binocular vision (after occlusion has achieved normal visual acuity in the squinting eye); others believe that this outcome is not often obtained and prefer to limit operations to cosmetic indications, for example shortly before the child starts school or in his/her early 'teens, if at all.

In giving you the history, a mother may say that her child 'squints' when she means that he merely 'screws up' (i.e. half-closes his eyes); make sure that she means that one eye turns inwards towards the nose, or outwards.

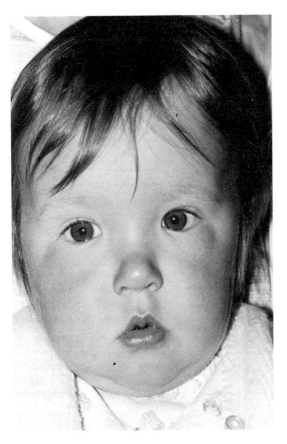

Fig 3.4 Epicanthic folds. This child *appears* to have a left convergent squint partly because of crescentic folds of skin at the inner angles (canthi) of the eyelids. Another reason is that the child is looking slightly to her right. The bright spots of light in the pupil areas ('corneal reflections') are reasonably central *and symmetrical* which strongly suggests the absence of squint. Cover test is negative.

Epicanthic folds

These are a common reason for a misdiagnosis of a convergent squint in a child. They are crescentic folds of skin at the inner canthus, which disappear as the bridge of the nose develops (Fig 3.4; *see also* Fig 12.6). To be sure that a squint is not present, use the cover/uncover test described below. The typical history of epicanthic folds in a young child is of a 'constant squint from birth'. Another typical history from an adult is that he had a squint as a child and later grew out of it; that never happens—the squint must have been only apparent and probably due to epicanthic folds.

The commonest cause of unilateral reduced visual acuity discovered incidentally or accidentally in a child or an adult with no previous symptoms is a small degree of squint along with strabismic amblyopia which has never previously been noticed. Again the diagnosis depends on the cover/uncover test.

Cover/uncover test (Fig 3.5)

The patient is asked to look at an object as far away as possible: adults and older children can look at, say, a specified part of the 6/60 letter on the test chart, a child of 3–4 years will look at a small picture of a bird or house on a fixation bar held in the examiner's hand, while a 2-year-old may be persuaded to fix on a flashing torchlight for long enough to allow the test to be done.

Suppose the child is suspected of a right concomitant convergent squint and we have excluded a right lateral rectus weakness by testing ocular movements. Having contrived to make the patient fix his gaze on a suitable fixation object, the examiner crisply covers the left eye with one hand but watches the right. If the right eye moves outwards to take up fixation, then the right had been convergent before the left was covered— i.e. the diagnosis of a right convergent squint is confirmed. If no movement of the right eye occurs, it has no squint (assuming it is not blind!). The examiner *uncovers* the left eye and moves the fixation object around a little to let the usual state re-establish itself. Then he crisply covers the right eye but watches the left. The left eye, already being consistently used for fixation, will not move. The right eye is then uncovered. Repeat the test several times if you are in doubt: watch each eye very carefully to detect the very small movement when a squint of very small angle is present. The test may be difficult—or impossible—in a 1½- to 2-year-old; depending on the strength of the history, review the patient in a week or so and then in a further few weeks.

Eccentric fixation

This is a not uncommon end-result of a long-standing unilateral squint,

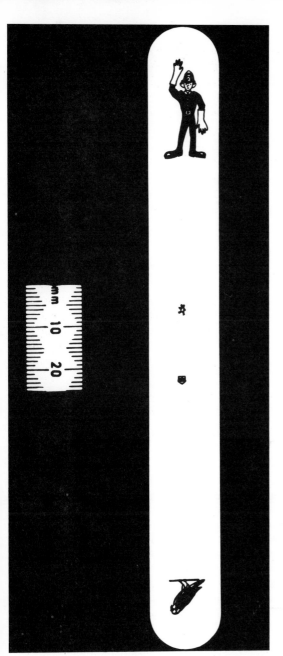

Fig 3.5 Cover test.
(a) Useful fixation objects for a 2- to 6-year-old child.

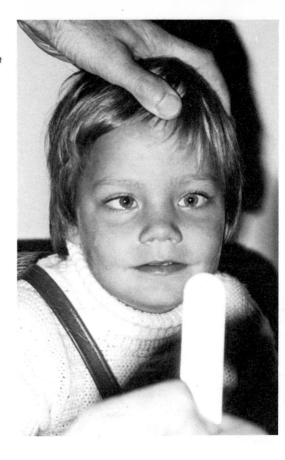

(b) Child looking at, say, a picture of a bird at the top of the white fixation bar held in the examiner's hand. The right convergent squint is obvious. Note that the bright spot of light (reflection from the cornea) in the left eye is near the centre of the pupil but on the right is nearer the lateral margin of the pupil because of the right convergence.

especially if it started in early life. Suppose the right eye is converged so that the image received at the *left* macula corresponds with an image received by the right retina at a point between the macula and the optic disc. Poor visual acuity (i.e. dense amblyopia at the right macula) occurs. However, the brain may reorientate the spatial values of the right retina, and accept the point between macula and disc as representing 'straight ahead', although acuity there is probably only 6/60. A cover test will now show no abnormality, but the patient has a definite squint! Occlusion of the left eye will do no good—the right eye will struggle to use its abnormal point of fixation as best it can. An ingenious diagnostic test is to use a small 'star' incorporated into the ophthalmoscope, and while you do ophthalmoscopy on the right eye (cover the left), ask the patient to 'look at the star'. The examiner will then see the point on the retina between disc and macula which the eye is using for eccentric fixation.

Treatment is usually only partially successful. The *eccentric* eye is covered for many weeks to try to make the retina 'forget' its abnormal spatial values,

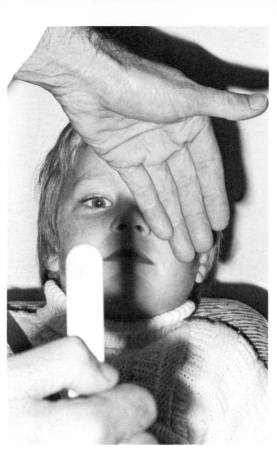

(c) The examiner crisply covers the left eye and observes that the right turns outwards to take up fixation— i.e. the right was converged before the left was covered, therefore there is a right convergent squint.

and then the good eye is covered in the hope that the amblyopia can be overcome.

Divergent

A concomitant divergent squint is unusual. It tends to present around the age of 7 or 8 years with a history that for several months one eye has glided outwards occasionally, especially when the child is tired. The child seldom complains of diplopia. It tends to progress throughout life. There is usually no significant refractive error and the cause is unknown. If or when the symptoms are troublesome or if the divergent squint is likely to become permanent, with loss of binocular single vision, a lateral rectus recession with or without medial rectus resection is required—and in future years the fellow eye may require operation.

A blind eye in an adult tends to diverge.

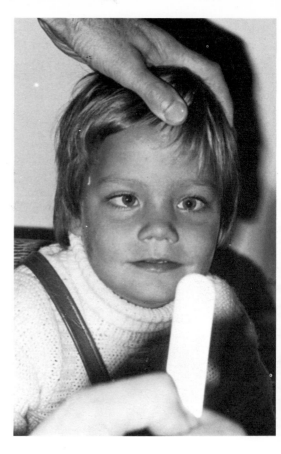

(d) The examiner *uncovers* the left eye and moves the fixation object around to let the eyes return to their usual state.

Value of binocular vision

There are very few occupations in which full stereoscopic vision is essential. Indeed, it is remarkable how well one-eyed patients manage—hence the varying attitude to binocularity on the part of ophthalmologists. Air pilots are usually required to have full stereoscopic vision. I reject candidates who wish to take up ophthalmic surgery unless they have full stereoscopic vision—as well as steady hands: both are particularly important in microsurgery, which is an integral part of ophthalmology. However, its importance in the generality of occupations and sports should not be overestimated.

Incomitant squint

As mentioned above, before a diagnosis of 'concomitant' squint is made,

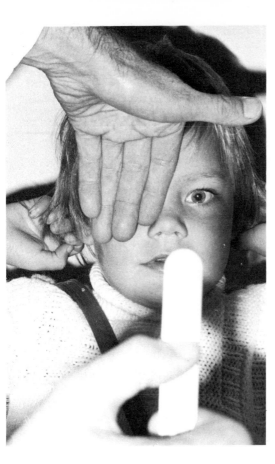

it is important to test ocular movements carefully—often in each eye separately, one being covered while the other is tested. To miss a lateral rectus paralysis due to an intracranial tumour in a young child may be disastrous: fortunately it is a rarity, just as incomitant squints in children in general are rare.

In an adult, an incomitant squint, whatever its cause, usually presents with diplopia. A young child will not have the vocabulary to complain of diplopia and anyway a child under, say, 4 years suppresses the image from one eye as soon as diplopia occurs. The diplopia will be horizontal if horizontal movements are affected (e.g. lateral rectus paralysis) or vertical with a tilt if a superior or inferior rectus muscle, or a superior or inferior oblique muscle is affected.

An elderly patient may compain of 'diplopia', when 'blurred vision' is meant, usually due to cataract. In case only blurred vision is the problem, *early in the history always ask the patient 'Does the double vision remain if you shut the right eye?'* and then *'Does the double vision remain if you shut the left eye?'*. If the answer to either or both of these questions is 'Yes' then *binocular* diplopia is *not* present, so the differential diagnosis relates to that of blurred vision in one or both eyes.

In a case of binocular diplopia (which disappears when either eye is shut) details should be elicited about total duration from its onset, how often and for how long it is present, whether it is horizontal or vertical or has a tilt, and whether the separation of images is greatest looking up, down, right or left. A detailed *general* history, especially regarding the CNS, is important.

Careful testing of ocular movements is essential but may reveal no abnormality to inspection in cases of a *weak* (not paralysed) extraocular muscle. Make the patient fix his gaze on your finger held in front of him and make him keep looking at that finger as you move it up, down, right and left, and to the intermediate points. Note that the superior oblique muscle (IVth nerve) depresses the adducted eye, so particular attention is paid to that movement in each eye. The VIth cranial nerve supplies the lateral rectus muscle. All other extraocular muscles (superior, inferior and medial recti, and inferior oblique) as well as the elevator muscle of the upper lid and the parasympathetic intraocular muscles (ciliary and sphincter pupillae) are supplied by the IIIrd cranial nerve.

If the observer cannot see any weakness of the patient's ocular movements, he should do an examination on the Hess chart or Hess screen. In principle, the patient wears goggles, a red glass in front of the right eye and a green glass in front of the left eye. He sits in front of a black screen which has a grid pattern on it, each intersection being marked by a red dot which can be seen only by the right eye. In one hand he holds a stick with a green ring at the end, or a torch with a green light, visible to his left eye only. Accordingly, the right and left eyes are dissociated—i.e. the red points on the screen are seen only by the right eye, the green ring or spot of light by the left eye. The examiner points to each red dot in turn and asks the patient to place his green ring/light exactly on it. The examiner records on a corresponding chart where the patient puts the green indicator, then at the end inspects the chart to discover the direction(s) of gaze in which the green spot falls short. For example, if there is a weakness of the left lateral rectus muscle, then when the patient is looking at the red dots on the screen to his left, the green indicator will be applied to a point less far to the left than it should be; to the right the green indicator will coincide with the red dots.

Diagnosis

The exact identification of an affected muscle or movement is often unnecessary for a diagnosis. It is a good plan to consider for the diagnosis, first, lesions in the orbit, and then work gradually backwards—

the neuromuscular junction, then muscle itself, then nerve lesions in the orbit, nerve lesions in the intracranial cavity, in the brain itself and finally the nerve nucleus. Lesions higher than the level of the nucleus produce gaze palsies and will be mentioned shortly.

The commonest orbital lesion producing diplopia is probably dysthyroid exophthalmos, usually with proptosis and upper lid retraction. Occasionally a lacrimal gland or other orbital tumour is a cause. Surprisingly, myasthenia gravis may be unilateral and have a sudden onset of diplopia, usually with ptosis, and may show no fluctuation in severity. A tensilon test usually confirms the diagnosis. Probably the commonest 'nerve' lesion is a congenital underaction which occasionally produces transient diplopia for several years with no other symptoms, especially when the patient is tired. Intracranial tumours are rare but important causes; for example, parasellar meningioma, pituitary tumour and craniopharyngioma.

A young adult presenting with diplopia of a few days' duration and no other symptoms, with no obvious weakness of ocular movements, quite probably has a localized demyelinating lesion due to multiple sclerosis: this is confirmed when the symptoms disappear slowly after 2–3–4–6 weeks, but of course there are quite likely to be serious implications in later life. The nerve supply of any muscle may be affected—lateral rectus (VI), superior oblique (IV), or any of the muscles supplied by the IIIrd nerve. An interesting and not uncommon problem is a selective weakness of convergence with or without accommodation after concussion, part of the IIIrd nerve nucleus being selectively affected; treatment is by base-in prisms with or without reading addition.

Treatment is that of the underlying condition, but prisms may be used in cases of recovering or slight permanent weakness—the apex of the prism pointing away from the direction of action of the weak muscle. Weight and cosmetic disadvantages prevent the use of thick prisms in severe or complete paralysis. Surgical treatment is possible: either the overacting antagonist muscle or the contralateral synergist is weakened by a recession.

Gaze palsies

A supranuclear lesion, anywhere between a point just higher than the nucleus up to the cerebral cortex, is rare but interesting in that it produces paralysis of gaze. The reason is that the affected supranuclear fibres carry 'orders' to both eyes, say, to look right, before these are translated by the nuclei into specific stimuli to different muscles on the two sides—in this example the right lateral rectus (VIth nerve) and the left medial rectus (part of IIIrd nerve). The commonest lesion is a cerebral thrombosis or a limited intracerebral haemorrhage, often associated with hemiparesis which makes the abnormality more difficult to detect.

Nystagmus

The commonest cause of this 'wobbling' movement of the eyes is *congenitally* poor vision in *both* eyes from whatever cause—cataract, foveal (macular) dysplasia, rubella retinopathy etc. Sometimes it is hereditary from some unknown lesion in the CNS, most commonly due to an X-linked recessive (or X-linked dominant) gene.

The next most common situation is in established multiple sclerosis, and it can be seen at the extremes of gaze. Ask the patient to watch your finger as you move it far to his left; stop near his furthest point of gaze and you will see his eyes drift slowly towards the centre, then jerk quickly back to fixation.

Physiological nystagmus occurs when you sit as a passenger in a railway train looking out of the window. It also arises after speedy rotation around the central axis of the body.

The subject is an interesting, very large and sometimes complicated one. Of course it overlaps considerably with neurology and otology.

Reference

1 Blakemore C and van Sluyters R C (1974) Experimental analysis of amblyopia and strabismus. *Br J Ophthalmol* **58**, 176–80

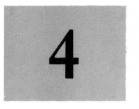

Refractive Errors, Spectacles and Contact Lenses

4

C I Phillips

Suggestions for teachers

It should be emphasized that refractive errors are not merely optical problems; for example, myopia is associated with retinal detachments and open-angle glaucoma, and hypermetropia with convergent squint and with angle-closure glaucoma.

To explain astigmatism it is useful to have constructed a simple model, using a Perspex dome as cornea slightly 'buckled' between two vertical props, and with black and white insulating wire to represent rays of light passing through holes in it.

A demonstration of a range of spectacles is useful and also gives the student time to absorb the teaching outside the usual tutorial times. Each pair of spectacles should have a card explaining whether it is a plus or minus lens and what refractive error it treats. Students can also learn the rudiments of neutralization as a means of estimating the power of a spectacle lens: put a trial lens of the opposite sign with the spectacle lens.

The normal eye: emmetropia (absence of a refractive error)

The normal adult eyeball has an axial length, from the front of the cornea to the posterior pole, of about 24 mm (Fig 4.1). However, there is a wide variance, as for human height, blood pressure etc., and so emmetropic eyes vary between 21 mm and 26 mm. By definition, the refracting system of an emmetropic eye, with accommodation relaxed, will bring parallel rays of light entering the pupil to a focus on the retina (i.e. within a very short distance). When an emmetropic eye has a short axial length, say 21 mm, Nature has compensated for that by making the cornea

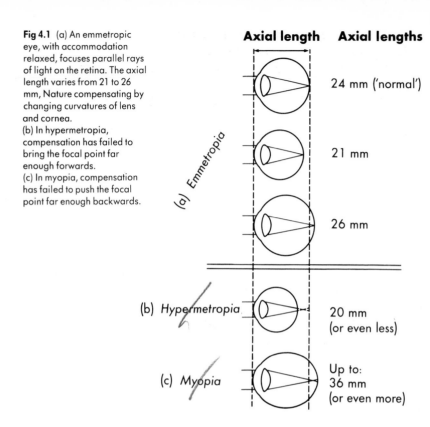

Fig 4.1 (a) An emmetropic eye, with accommodation relaxed, focuses parallel rays of light on the retina. The axial length varies from 21 to 26 mm, Nature compensating by changing curvatures of lens and cornea.
(b) In hypermetropia, compensation has failed to bring the focal point far enough forwards.
(c) In myopia, compensation has failed to push the focal point far enough backwards.

Axial length

Axial lengths

24 mm ('normal')

21 mm

26 mm

(a) Emmetropia

(b) Hypermetropia

20 mm
(or even less)

(c) Myopia

Up to:
36 mm
(or even more)

and the surfaces of the crystalline lens steeper in curvature than in a 24 mm eye. Similarly, continuing the teleological principle, if an emmetropic eyeball has an axial length of 26, Nature must have compensated by producing less convex surfaces of the cornea and crystalline lens. Surveys have been done in which optical methods have been used to measure the dioptric powers of cornea and lens, and ultrasound for axial length, hence these accurate statistics.

The most powerful refractive component of the eye, of course, is the interface between air and *anterior* corneal surface since these two differ most in refractive index. The corneal surface is convex towards air so that parallel rays passing from air to cornea are converged. (The *diverging* effect of the posterior surface of cornea is much less because the refractive index of aqueous humour is only slightly different from that of cornea.)

The net refractive power of the cornea is around 43 dioptres. Both surfaces of the crystalline lens produce convergence of rays of light because the refractive index of the lens is greater than that of aqueous and vitreous humour. Furthermore, the refractive index of lens increases towards its centre, so that more convergence of rays of light can be achieved. The power of the crystalline lens is around 17 dioptres. Contraction of the ciliary muscle, however, *slackens* the suspensory ligament of the lens which then indulges its natural tendency to get fatter—i.e. increases the curvatures of its surfaces (called 'accommodation'). At around 8 years, accommodation can add about 14 dioptres of dioptic power, and it is presumably even higher in younger children. However, it declines progressively with increasing age until at around 65 years it is usually zero.

Presbyopia

By about 45 years in Caucasians and about 35 years often in other races, accommodation can add only about 3D to the power of the eye. Since print is usually held at a distance of 0.33 metre from the eye, at these ages the full power of available accommodation is required but tiring will often occur with blurred vision and sometimes aching in the eyes. The need to use spectacles for near or close work then arises (*see* Chapter 2).

Hypermetropia (*see also* Chapter 3)

Hypermetropia (= hyperopia in USA) or long-sightedness usually arises from a relatively short axial length, as low as 19 or 20 mm, for which the dioptric power of cornea and lens have not been modified enough to compensate (Fig 4.1). Most cases are of low degree. Accommodation of around two or three dioptres can be constantly exerted even for distance vision without symptoms until about 35 years of age. Eventually, there is an earlier than usual onset of presbyopia. However, in some cases the convergence which is closely geared to accommodation produces a convergent squint. In more marked hypermetropia, a child or young adult may have blurred vision for near and also for distance.

Complications

In addition to a predisposition to a convergent squint, hypermetropia is also associated with angle-closure glaucoma which occurs usually over the age of 50 years (*see* Chapter 5).

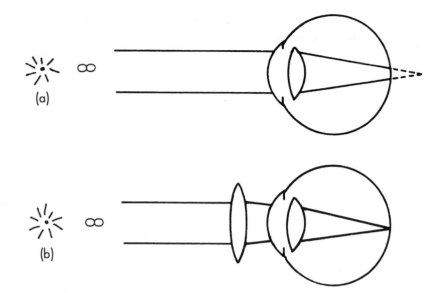

Fig 4.2 Hypermetropic eye, with short axial length.

(a) Parallel rays of light from an infinitely distant spot produce a blurred image on retina.

(b) A biconvex (+) spectacle lens converges the rays slightly before the eye's refracting system imposes the remainder of the vergence.

Treatment

When there are significant symptoms, a convex (+) spectacle lens is used even for distance vision (Fig 4.2).

Myopia

The usual cause of myopia is an axial length which is long in relation to the refractive power of cornea and lens, even though Nature has contrived to reduce the curvatures of cornea and lens (*see* Fig 4.1). Onset is around 7 or 8 years when distance vision is blurred: the child cannot see the writing on the blackboard. However, he can see to read quite easily with reduced accommodation, or none at all, if and when his myopia becomes severe enough. The disease tends to progress for a variable number of years, with an annual increase in strength of spectacle lenses. The cause is unknown in most cases but, in some, excessive close work and/or heredity may play a part. It is not known whether the abnormal size of eyeball results from some unknown stimulus to growth of sclera with resulting overstretching of retina (which seems likely) or vice versa—or some other unknown cause. Not surprisingly, it results from raised intraocular pressure in congenital glaucoma. Amazingly, tarsorrhaphy* in newborn monkeys will produce myopia after a year or so [1]; likewise ptosis or corneal or lens opacities may produce it in children [2]. In the elderly, early cataract with increased refractive index of the nucleus of the lens may present with myopia. Similarly in diabetics, but their refractive error often varies by several dioptres on different days as the blood sugar level varies.

Complications

These explain why myopes, especially those with more than −10D, constitute a higher proportion of the blind than emmetropes and hypermetropes. The 'high myope' (usually over −10D dioptres) in middle or later life may develop chorioretinal atrophy at the posterior pole with central scotomata; scotomata may occur quite suddenly because of subretinal or retinal haemorrhages at the macula. Both may be attributed to a lifetime of overstretching of the retina, but that is an oversimplification. Retinal detachments tend to occur in myopes because (1) peripheral retinal patches of degeneration become fixedly attached to vitreous so that when (2) vitreous degeneration and collapse occur (as they tend to do earlier in life in myopes than in others), the mobile vitreous tugs on these spots of retina, especially superiorly of course, and produces a round hole or arrowhead tear. Fluid then passes through the retinal hole to detach the retina progressively. If the hole in the retina is produced at the site of a retinal blood vessel, the latter may be torn and pour blood into the vitreous cavity — the patient sees a sudden heavy snowstorm of 'floating spots'.

Myopes tend to have a higher intraocular pressure than do emmetropes, which is probably why there is an unexpectedly high proportion of patients with myopia amongst those with chronic simple glaucoma. Raised intraocular pressure may be a causative factor in myopia — or may result from it.

The stronger the spectacle lens (*see* below) used to treat this disease, the more the peripheral field of vision is constricted, partly because of the prismatic effect of the periphery of concave lenses, and also because of the actual blocking of rays at the rims of the lenses, aggravated by frames.

Treatment

Optical treatment of myopia consists of prescribing concave lenses of appropriate power (Fig 4.3). Unlike hypermetropia, which tends to

---

* Tarsorrhaphy means stitching together the rawed lid margins so that they fuse.

remain stationary throughout life, myopia tends to progress so that changes in spectacles annually, or even more frequently, may be required until progression ceases — usually when growth in height stops. Breakage of concave (minus) lenses is quite common because the centres are thin, and they are often worn by children. Accordingly, plastic lenses or 'toughened glass' lenses should be prescribed to prevent accidental damage to the eyeball from broken glass. The higher the myopia the more the optical (and cosmetic) benefit from contact lenses.

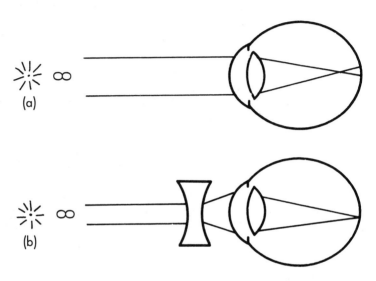

Fig 4.3 Myopic eye with long axial length.

(a) Parallel rays of light are brought to a focus in front of the retina so that a point source at infinity produces a blurred image on the retina.

(b) A biconcave (−) spectacle lens diverges the rays so that the refracting system of the eye converges the rays to a point image on the retina.

    Surgical treatment of myopia is being done in some centres: radial keratotomy. About a dozen or so deep radiating incisions are made outwards from a point about 2 mm from the centre of the cornea for a distance of about 3 mm, which causes a flattening of the curvature of the central area of cornea. Other surgical treatments for high myopia — shortening of the axial length by excision of a strip of sclera 3–4 mm broad from all round the equator of the eyeball with suturing of the edges, or removal of the crystalline lens (as in cataract extractions) — are no longer done.

Astigmatism

1. Regular

Superimposed on myopia or hypermetropia, or independently of either, there may be regular 'astigmatism' which is almost invariably due to a congenital distortion of the cornea (Fig 4.4). The normal cornea can be regarded optically as part of the wall of a transparent hollow sphere. In astigmatism, one meridian, say the vertical (i.e. from 12 to 6 o'clock), may be more or less convex than the one at right angles to it. Imagine a short section of the wall of the inner tube of a bicycle tyre: in the plane of the wheel, the curvature is much flatter than at right angles to that plane. Any meridians may be affected but always at right angles to each other. The result is that a point source of light at infinity cannot produce a point image on the retina ('astigmatism' comes from Greek: *a*, not; *stigma*, a point).

Treatment
Treatment of regular astigmatism is by an astigmatic spectacle lens (Fig 4.4).

Because the disease is congenital, and not severe, presenting symptoms are usually subnormal visual acuity discovered at the first school eye test around 6 years of age: the child with two to three dioptres of astigmatism does not realize that his visual acuity is only about 6/12 until he meets school work.

Small degrees of hypermetropia, myopia and astigmatism, especially if unilateral, do not require correction by spectacles or contact lenses.

2. Irregular astigmatism

This is rare. The surface of the cornea is uneven so that rays of light impinging on the surface are scattered in all directions as they pass through. The commonest cause is injury, the effect being usually unilateral. A corneal dystrophy, epithelial or endothelial, may cause it, but these are rare; the least rare is keratoconus in which the central area of the cornea becomes thin in late adolescence and protrudes forwards irregularly, with or without some opacification. There are many forms of corneal dystrophy, most of them hereditary, and almost all bilateral.

Treatment
Treatment of irregular astigmatism is by a contact lens which traps tears between the lens and cornea. Since the refractive index of tears is

Fig 4.4 Mixed astigmatism—i.e. one meridian myopic and the other, at right angles, hypermetropic. For the uncorrected eye, imagine a combination of diagrams (a) and (c).

(a) Parallel rays from an infinitely distant point object in the plane of the paper will produce a real point image in front of the retina and a vertical line actually on the retina. This meridian is myopic. (Note. The vertical bars in the diagram indicate the breadth of the beam of light, and should not be confused with the parallel rays of light from infinity.)

(b) A concave cylindrical lens diverges these rays to produce a point image on the retina. Note that in the plane at right angles to the paper this lens has no refractive power.

(c) Parallel rays from an infinitely distant object in a plane *at right angles* to the paper would produce an image behind the retina, but a horizontal line on the retina. This meridian is hyper-metropic.

(d) A convex cylindrical lens converges these rays to produce a point image on the retina. Note that in the plane of the paper (i.e. at right angles to the plane in which these rays exist) this lens has no refractive power.

To treat this state of 'mixed' astigmatism, a lens with these two properties would be used, the front surface convex horizontally and the back surface concave vertically.

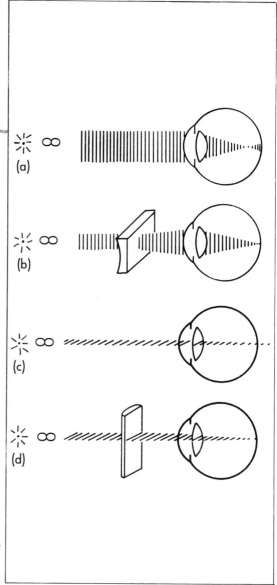

practically the same as cornea and contact lens, the refractive effect of the irregular anterior corneal surface is eliminated, being replaced by the smooth regular anterior surface of the contact lens. However, it may be that accompanying corneal opacities also scatter or block rays, reducing the effectiveness of the contact lens. In that case a corneal graft may be required.

Unilateral refractive errors

It is appropriate here to discuss treatment of patients with one emmetropic eye and one ametropic eye. This is a special case of anisometropia, a condition of unequal refraction in the right and left eyes. Many patients with one normal and one ametropic eye notice no disability throughout life, and indeed may only become aware of the poor vision in the affected eye accidentally at any age, or merely incidentally at a school eye test. For them, binocular vision is of little importance.

Ophthalmologists vary in their attitude to treatment of unilateral refractive errors, some prescribing spectacles or a contact lens because of some improvement in the overall visual state (especially field) and often the achievement of binocular vision; others prefer to avoid the disadvantages of spectacles and risks of a contact lens and the expense of both especially because many patients find the small optical advantages not worth the nuisance of these optical aids, and abandon them after a few months or years. Probably few ophthalmologists recommend a corneal graft for unilateral corneal opacities because of the risks, general and local, of operations and the possibility of a host–graft reaction.

Deprivation amblyopia

If a child has congenital *unilateral* hypermetropia or astigmatism without squint, the other eye being approximately emmetropic or less ametropic, the visual acuity in the more abnormal eye will be somewhat reduced— 'anisometropic amblyopia'—even when correcting spectacles are used. Improvement to normal can be achieved by the constant wearing of spectacles and intermittent occlusion of the good eye provided that this is done before the age of about 10 or 11 years (*strabismic* amblyopia should not be treated by occlusion after the age of about 6 or 7 years).

Congenital *unilateral* cataract or corneal opacity produces an extreme form of deprivation amblyopia. Congenital *bilateral* cataract or corneal opacity also produces deprivation amblyopia, but it is *less* dense than in unilateral cases.

Contact lenses

The most commonly used type are made of polymethylmethacrylate ('acrylic') and have a diameter of 10–11 mm so that they sit or swim around on the cornea. They are hard and slightly brittle. Their back curve is slightly steeper than that of the anterior surface of the cornea: the curvature of the front surface can be chosen to correct the patient's refractive error—in myopes, it will be less steep than that of the anterior corneal surface. 'Soft' contact lenses are made of polyhema (hydroxy-ethylmethacrylate, or one of its co-polymers) and are often tolerated better than the hard ones. There are also much larger 'scleral haptic' lenses, with a diameter more than 2.5 cm, which are very occasionally indicated in, for example, steep keratoconous or to hold drugs in contact with the cornea in high concentration.

All patients naturally feel some discomfort like that caused by foreign body when they start to wear them. Many learn to tolerate them remarkably quickly but a few never do.

Sterilization of hard contact lenses is by chemical solutions. Soft lenses are more difficult to sterilize than hard lenses, because of their spongy structure, and are usually boiled. Patients should be taught to handle their lenses with as near sterile precautions as possible.

The majority of contact lenses are worn to treat myopia, particularly to eliminate the constriction of the peripheral field produced by spectacles in myopia of more than around −10 dioptres. Progressively below that level, the optical indication becomes less strong and the cosmetic more important—especially for women who often prefer to avoid wearing spectacles. They are particularly useful in many cases of irregular astigmatism, and may allow the patient to avoid a corneal graft.

Contraindications are in patients who cannot learn to tolerate these 'foreign bodies' (asthmatics and allergics are often in that category) or who do not have the manual dexterity to cope with them (e.g. many of the elderly).

Complications of wearing them include corneal abrasions which may become infected to become corneal ulcers. Fortunately, the latter are rare but they can be disastrous, leading to total loss of vision or even of the eye itself, hence the need for unremitting maximum hygienic precautions.

Corneal grafts

A central superficial unvascularized corneal opacity is ideal for a *partial-thickness (lamellar)* corneal graft. (Let us ignore the question of whether the patient's other eye is normal or not.) A corneal trephine with a diameter just greater than that of the opacity, usually 5, 6, 7 or 8 mm, is applied to the cornea and rotated; the central plunger is set to allow the trephine to cut, say, only three-quarters of the way through the cornea. The superficial lamella containing the opacity is then dissected off (an operation microscope is more than useful for this) and discarded. A donor disc is trephined and dissected from a healthy donor eye, preferably of the same tissue type as the recipient's. The healthy disc is then sutured into place with fine needles and sutures. If the recipient cornea is vascularized (e.g. following a corneal ulcer), a graft–host reaction is much more likely because invisible lymphatics also accompany the visible blood vessels. Otherwise the operation is relatively safe, apart from the usual hazards of general anaesthesia and infection; but inadvertent penetration too deeply into the anterior chamber is a serious complication.

If the corneal opacity is deeper, then a *full-thickness* disc of cornea, usually 5, 6, 7 or 8 mm in diameter, has to be removed and replaced by a similar full-thickness disc from a donor eye which is sutured into place. More complications are likely than in a partial-thickness graft; for example, adhesion between the iris and the edge of the graft (the anterior chamber is flat at operation and for a few hours thereafter), and tilting of the graft (with optical effects) as well as the usual danger of rejection especially if the host cornea is vascularized.

Pin-hole test

This simple test is valuable for the non-ophthalmologist to find out if a patient's reduced visual acuity is due to a refractive error (even irregular corneal astigmatism) or not. If you have mislaid that essential piece of equipment, a black disc with a small 0.5 mm diameter central hole, a thick pin can be used to pierce an appropriate hole in a thin piece of card or paper. The hole should be held as close as possible to the patient's eye, thus eliminating most of the effect of its lens system. (A pin-hole camera will produce an image without *any* lens system!) An improvement in the patient's acuity of several lines on the test chart supports the diagnosis of refractive error, especially if 6/6 is achieved. No improvement will occur in cataract, macular degeneration, optic atrophy etc.

Refraction

In order to decide whether or not a patient has a refractive error, the ophthalmologist or optician performs a 'refraction'. There are two stages, and the student should see this being done in the outpatient department and obtain an explanation. A full account is inappropriate in this book, but the following outline should suffice.

In stage 1, a retinoscopy or skiascopy is done—an 'objective' method in so far as minimal co-operation is required from the patient. A spot or streak of light is shone through the pupil of the patient's eye from an instrument like a direct ophthalmoscope to illuminate an area of retina. Then the light is moved up, down, right and left (or obliquely if oblique astigmatism is present), which moves the illuminated area on the retina up, down, right and left respectively. The illuminated area of retina sends rays of light back through the patient's pupil to form an image: depending on the refractive error, the position of the image (i.e. its plane) will vary. To the observer, the direction of movement of the image may well *not* be the same as the direction of movement which he knows he has imposed on the light he is shining on to the retina. Accordingly, he can differentiate refractive errors into myopia and hypermetropia and astigmatism. He then chooses the appropriate series of lenses to place in a trial frame on the patient's face with the aim of *reversing* the direction of movement of the light: by trial and error he increases the strength of these trial lenses until reversal of movement occurs, which lens indicates the amount of refractive error present. If the reversing lens is different in two meridians, the difference between the two indicates the amount of astigmatism present.

Stage 2 is the 'subjective' part—i.e. the patient helps to estimate more precisely the spectacle correction which has been predicted fairly accurately from stage 1. The ophthalmologist tests the right eye first and then the left, blocking vision in one eye with a black disc. He places a lens in the trial frame and establishes how far down the test chart (Snellen's: for distance) the patient can read. He then varies the power of the spheres and cylinders in the trial frame, and alters the axis of the cylinder until maximum improvement in visual acuity is achieved—up to 6/6 in normal eyes.

In young children, and mental defectives, stage 2 is impossible, so spectacles have to be prescribed after stage 1. For stage 1, in order to eliminate variations in accommodation in the 6-year-old and younger, homatropine 1% eyedrops are instilled into both eyes an hour before the appointment—by mother, at home: in dark-skinned races atropine 1% eyedrops may be necessary in the under-6-year-old.

'Diagnosis' of unknown spectacle lenses

If the lenses in a pair of spectacles are unknown, it is possible to determine the power. This is most quickly and accurately done with a focimeter, which is standard equipment in all eye clinics. However, a non-specialist can obtain a lot of information from inspection and palpation!

A practical demonstration plus a little practice in the outpatient department will be easier to understand than the following account.

Hold the unknown lenses close to your eyes (turn the spectacle legs away from you) and look through the lens at a distant object. If the object looks smaller, the spectacle lens is concave (−): the patient's eye is myopic. If the object merely looks blurred, and possibly bigger, the lens is a convex (+) lens: the patient's eye is hypermetropic. Move the lens a very short way up and down and side to side: if the object appears to move in the same direction as the movement of the lens, the lens is concave (−); if the object moves in the opposite direction, the lens is convex (+).

To detect an astigmatic lens, again hold the lens quite close to your eye, the legs away from you, but position it so that you can see a vertical or horizontal line in the distance (e.g. a corner of the room) both through the lens *and* outside it. Position the lens (if necessary, rotate it) so that the line viewed outside and inside the lens is continuous and unbroken. Then rotate the lens: if the line viewed through the lens also rotates to an oblique position (i.e. there is an angle of less than 180 degrees between it and the line outside the lens) then there is an astigmatic correction in that lens.

A strong concave lens can also be detected because its thick edge and thinner centre are obvious to inspection and touch. A strong convex lens (e.g. used after cataract extraction) has a thicker centre than periphery.

Strength of an 'unknown' spectacle lens

The property of apparent movement can be used to estimate the power of the lens. For example, if you have decided a lens is *convex*, with some astigmatism, take from a lens box a *concave* lens, hold it concentric, and in contact, with the unknown and move the combined pair: if any apparent movement remains, try another lens (stronger concave if the movement is still opposite, less strong if the movement has been changed to 'with'). Keep trying until no movement whatsoever is obtained in one meridian of movement—the value of the neutralizing lens gives the strength of the sphere. Proceed to 'neutralize' the movement in the other meridian, and the difference between the two neutralizing lenses gives the amount of the cylinder.

Prisms

A prism is so rarely incorporated into a spectacle lens (e.g. in treatment of a squint) that this slight complication need not be considered.

Lens prescriptions

With a little practice, the various ways in which these are presented can be interpreted easily. If a form is used with a box labelled 'sphere' and 'cylinder', the interpretation is easy. There is usually a box also for angle of cylinder, or a diagram like half of a compass card on which an arrow has been written to indicate that angle if a cylinder is present.

The clearest way to write a lens prescription is in the form of a fraction, the sphere above and the cylinder below the line, with visual acuity beside it, thus

$$\frac{-1.00}{0}^{R} : 6/6 \qquad \frac{0}{+3.00_{\downarrow 90°}}^{L} : 6/12$$

This means that the right eye achieves 6/6 visual acuity with a -1D sphere (no cylinder) but the left achieves only 6/12 with $+3.00$D cylinder at 90 degrees (no sphere). This patient has anisometropic amblyopia in his left eye. Another way of writing the above is:

$$-1DS\ (6/6) \qquad +3DC_{\times 90°}\ (6/12)$$

A further way, used less nowadays, is to put the information about the right eye on a line above the left: for example:

$$R\ -1DS\ (6/6)$$
$$L\ +3DC_{\times 90°}(6/12)$$

References

1 Wiesel T N and Raviola F (1977) Myopia and eye enlargement after neonatal lid fusion in monkeys. *Nature* **266**, 66–8
2 O'Leary D J and Millodot M (1978) Eyelid closure causes myopia in humans. *Experientia* **35**, 1478–9

5

Glaucoma

C I Phillips

Definition

'Glaucoma' occurs when an eye has an abnormally high intraocular
pressure. The average (mean) normal intraocular pressure is 16 mmHg
above atmospheric and its standard deviation is 2.6, because the variation
is quite wide. It is a quite fascinating property of the Gaussian or 'normal'
distribution curve of *any* biological quantity that the mean ±2 standard
deviations (SD) includes 95% of all the observations in that population
while ±3 SD includes 99.7%. Accordingly, one criterion of 'abnormally
high' intraocular pressure would be 16 mm + 2 SD (i.e.
16 mm + 2 × 2.6 = 21.2 mmHg) but the criterion usually applied in the
clinic is 16 mm + 3 SD (i.e. 16 mm + 3 × 2.6 = 23.8 ≏ 24 mmHg). Similar
considerations are already familiar in relation to blood pressure. Even
these criteria have to be applied with judgement because variations of
intraocular pressure (IOP) occur during 24 hours ('diurnal variation') and
the average pressure rises with age, as with blood pressure and quite
probably intracranial pressure: all three share many common properties.

Physiopathology

Aqueous humour is fundamental to the health of the eye, especially the
lens. All cases of glaucoma are due to reduced drainage of aqueous
humour but the cause is different in the four categories. Glaucoma is
never due to abnormally increased production of aqueous humour.

Aqueous humour is secreted by the ciliary epithelium—about 2–3 mm³
(microlitres, μl) per minute (*see* Plate 5.1). Very little diffuses posteriorly
through the vitreous to escape through the optic disc and retina. Almost
all flows slowly round the lens, passing through the struts of the

suspensory ligament, to arrive behind the iris. Then it passes through the pupil into the anterior chamber. From the angle of the anterior chamber, it passes through the *trabecular meshwork* into the *canal of Schlemm* and from there it goes via collector channels through the anterior sclera to reach the surface of the eyeball and join the subconjunctival veins. With the slit-lamp microscope, you *can* see 'aqueous veins' underneath conjunctiva near the limbus (corneoscleral junction). They contain clear fluid and join with blood-containing subconjunctival veins; the two streams run separately for some distance in the same vein—as do the two rivers the Blue and the White Nile.

Cerebrospinal fluid has a similar circulation. It is secreted by the choroid plexuses (like ciliary epithelium) in the lateral ventricles, from which it passes into the third ventricle, then into the aqueduct of Sylvius and fourth ventricle, and then through the foramina in its roof (analogous to the pupil) into the subarachnoid space.

The trabecular meshwork normally provides just the correct amount of resistance to outflow of aqueous, in relation to the amount secreted, to maintain intraocular pressure normal. It achieves this at the continuous layer of endothelium next to the canal of Schlemm (Fig 5.1). This layer engulfs droplets on the 'anterior chamber' side and passes them out into the canal of Schlemm. These droplets can be seen by the light microscope. The process is pressure-dependent—i.e. the number and/or rate of passage of droplets through the endothelial meshwork increases when intraocular pressure rises, and diminishes when pressure falls.

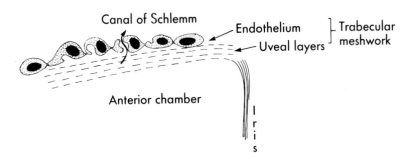

Fig 5.1 Diagram of cross-section of the top (12 o'clock) of the angle of the anterior chamber at the periphery of the iris, cornea being to left and sclera to right. The uveal layers of the trabecular meshwork provide very little resistance to the outflow of aqueous humour from the anterior chamber to the canal of Schlemm. The single layer of endothelial cells of the trabecular meshwork 'ingests' on one side, and 'excretes' at the other, droplets of aqueous humour to maintain outflow at the same rate as inflow in the normal eye. The cycle is shown from left to right, the arrow in a central cell indicating a through-and-through stage. (Adapted from Tripathi R C (1971) Mechanism of aqueous outflow across the trabecular wall of Schlemm's canal. *Exp Eye Res.* **11**, 116–21)

Unfortunately, there is no significant feedback mechanism which reduces secretion when the outflow mechanism is defective.

Again, it is extremely interesting to note that the analogy between cerebrospinal fluid and aqueous is close, because the surface of the arachnoid villi contains cells which probably deal with CSF in the same way as do the cells of the endothelial meshwork.

Special methods of examination in glaucoma

Tonometry

1. Applanation tonometry
This is frequently performed in eye clinics, as often as blood pressure in medical clinics. The best way to understand it is to see it being done, with explanation, or to do it oneself as in every clinical situation.

The principle is ingeniously simple (Fig 5.2), and the test is done without any discomfort to the patient following a drop or two of topical local anaesthetic, usually oxybuprocaine (benoxinate), to anaesthetize the cornea. A drop of fluorescein is then added and diffuses through the tears. If a flat plate is gently pressed against the cornea with a standard

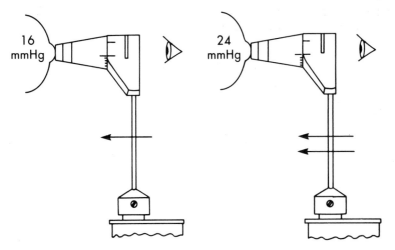

Fig 5.2 Applanation tonometry. When the intraocular pressure is 'normal' (16 mmHg) a certain amount of force (←) has to be applied to the applanation 'prism' touching the cornea to flatten a standard area of cornea. That area can be estimated easily by the tonometrist. When the pressure has reached the glaucoma range (24 mmHg and above), a greater force (⇄) is required to flatten the standard area. The force (in grams weight which ×10 gives mmHg) is read off a scale on the milled knob with which the tonometrist controls the force.

pressure, then the area of cornea flattened will be large if the intraocular pressure (IOP) is low, but the area will be small if the IOP is high. Similarly, if we can apply different pressures to the flat plate in order to achieve flattening of a *standard area of corneal surface*, then the pressure applied will have to be high when the intraocular pressure is high, whereas the pressure applied need only be slight when the pressure is low. The applanating 'prism' is situated at the end of an arm projecting vertically upwards from a 'black box' (Fig 5.3). A serrated knob on the outside of the box actuates a spring-loaded device which allows the tonometrist to increase or decrease the pressure exerted on the cornea by the plastic applanation 'prism'. The black box plus arm plus applanation 'prism' is mounted on the slit-lamp microscope (Fig 5.3) in such a way that the observer, looking through the eyepieces has a magnified view of the two half-rings (*see* Plate 5.2). The end-point, when the standard area of cornea has been cleared of fluorescein solution, is reached when the inner, rather indistinct, edges of the two half-rings are continuous.

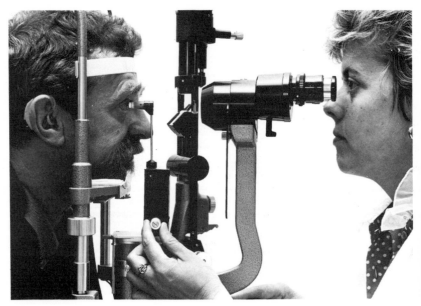

Fig 5.3 Applanation tonometry. (*See* Fig 5.2 for principles.) One end of the applanation 'prism' is in contact with the patient's anaesthetized cornea. The tonometrist obtains a magnified view through the eyepieces of the slit-lamp microscope of the flat end of the applanation prism which flattens a standard small area of the patient's cornea. The force on the prism, transmitted through the lever to which it is attached, is accurately controlled by the tonometrist's fingers rotating the milled knob.

There is an excellent hand-held version of the applanation tonometer which can be used independently of the slit-lamp microscope—for example, in the operation theatre or on a bed-fast patient.

The student will be interested to see the striking pulsation of the eyeball (i.e. the large swing of IOP with each pulse beat), as in intracranial pressure, which is obvious during tonometry.

2. Schiøtz tonometer

This instrument has been almost completely superseded by the applanation tonometer because the latter is more accurate under most circumstances. The Schiøtz tonometer depends on *indentation* of the (anaesthetized) cornea, as distinct from applanation. The principle is shown in Fig 5.4. If the intraocular pressure is high, the plunger can indent the cornea only slightly, and the pointer moves only a short distance along the scale. If the intraocular pressure is low, the plunger indents the cornea much more and the pointer moves a much greater distance across the scale. A calibration curve converts the scale reading into mmHg.

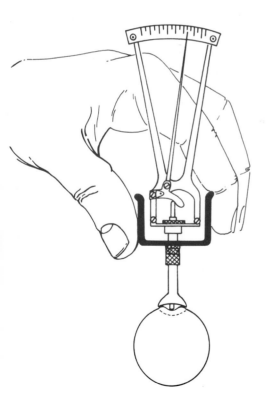

Fig 5.4 A Schiøtz tonometer is shown held by the tonometrist so that the footplate sits on the anaesthetized cornea (causing only minor discomfort). The lower end of the plunger of the instrument, emerging from the footplate, will indent the cornea— deeply if the intraocular pressure is low (as shown), very little if the pressure is high. The depth of indentation is magnified by a lever, and transmitted to a pointer which is backed by a scale in arbitrary units at the top of the picture. A calibration curve is available to convert these arbitrary units of indentation into mmHg.

The calibration curve was obtained from enucleated eyeballs of normal size and is required because, in the process of Schiøtz tonometry, the indentation raises the intraocular pressure considerably. If the eyeball in the patient is small (probably hypermetropic) the Schiøtz tonometer gives an erroneously high reading; if the eyeball is large, the reading will be erroneously low. The applanation tonometer suffers negligibly from this fault mainly because in the process of applanation the IOP is raised only 2–3 mmHg.

3. Digital tonometry
This is of limited value because even experienced fingers can distinguish only very high and very low intraocular pressure from the normal range through the closed eyelids (Fig 5.5). The test is very like that for 'fluctuation' in an abscess and the finger-pressure is very gentle.

Gonioscopy

The differentiation between open-angle and angle-closure glaucoma is vitally important (see below). The ophthalmologist must obtain a

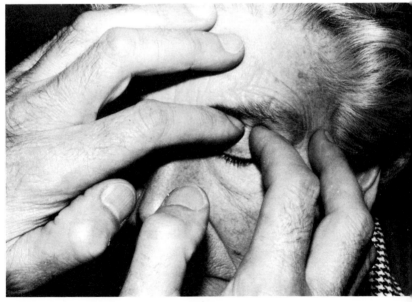

Fig 5.5 Digital tonometry. The patient is asked to close his eyes and look downwards. The tonometrist places his right and left index fingers on the lid over the eyeball, steadying his hands by placing the remaining fingers on the patient's forehead and temple. The left and right index fingers are alternately *gently* depressed into the eyeball to allow the eyeball to be classified into hard, soft or normal.

magnified view of the angle of the anterior chamber in every case. Unfortunately, rays of light coming out from the angle of the anterior chamber strike the cornea/air interface so obliquely that they are reflected back into the anterior chamber (Fig 5.6). To allow them to escape, a contact lens with a steeper curve than that of the cornea has to be placed over the (anaesthetized) cornea, with a layer of saline in the gap between the two. The refractive indices of cornea, saline and contact lens are very similar.

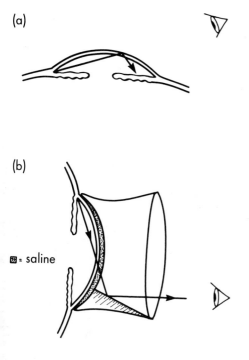

(a)

(b)

🔲 = saline

Fig 5.6 Gonioscopy. (a) An observer looking obliquely towards the angle of the anterior chamber is unable to see it because rays of light coming from the angle are totally internally reflected at the cornea/air interface. (b) Because the refractive indices of cornea, saline and Perspex are all similar, a contact lens with a steeper curve than cornea, and with saline between the two, will allow rays of light to pass through the corneal surface. The mirror is of minor importance and reflects rays of light forwards (patient sitting) for the convenience of the observer looking through his slit-lamp microscope (not shown in diagram).

The special contact lens used is called a gonioscopy lens, and often incorporates a mirror to reflect the rays of light forwards for the convenience of the examiner behind his slit-lamp microscope (Fig 5.7). The slit-lamp has a powerful focused light (which can be adjusted to a slit beam) on a movable arm and is integral with a microscope which also moves on an arm concentrically with the slit-lamp. (The student will be fascinated to see the quite beautiful detail that can be obtained with this instrument.)

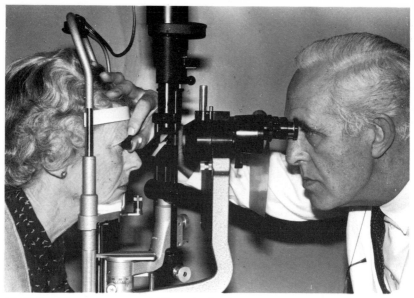

Fig 5.7 Gonioscopy.

(a) The patient has the gonioscope applied to her right eye following topical anaesthetic eyedrops. The observer sees a magnified stereoscopic view of the angle of the anterior chamber through the eyepieces of the slit-lamp microscope.

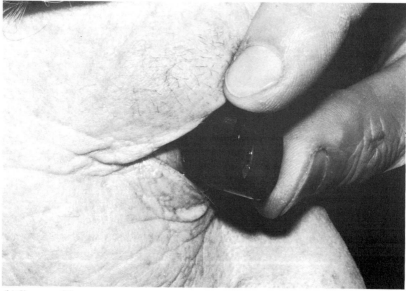

(b) Close-up of the gonioscope applied to the patient's right eye.

Classification

The subject will be considered under four headings:

1 Congenital or infantile glaucoma (buphthalmos)
2 Angle-closure glaucoma
3 Open-angle (chronic simple) glaucoma
4 Glaucoma due to iridocyclitis, neovascularization of the angle etc.,
  often called 'secondary' glaucoma

(Note. The first three are often called the 'primary' glaucomas—
unfortunately, because a great deal is known and accepted about their
causation.)

Congenital or infantile glaucoma (buphthalmos)

Cause
During intrauterine development, the anterior chamber is full of
mesoderm. Normally, by the time of birth this has disappeared, so that
aqueous humour secreted by the ciliary epithelium can escape. Very
rarely, this mesoderm fails to disappear completely and a residue remains
in the angle and obstructs the outflow of aqueous humour. Autosomal
recessive genes cause the disease, although males are more often affected
than females. The disease is usually bilateral, occasionally unilateral.

Symptoms and signs
Within a few weeks, or several months, from birth, the effects of the rise
in intraocular pressure become manifest. *The whole eyeball enlarges,*
hence 'buphthalmos'—Greek for the eye of an ox. (Note. After the age
of $2\frac{1}{2}$ years or so, raised intraocular pressure can no longer cause
dilatation of the eyeball, presumably because of maturation of its collagen
fibres.) Tears occur in the deepest layers of the cornea, Descemet's
membrane and the endothelium, so that some aqueous enters the cornea
to cause patches of oedema which appear grey–white to the examiner.
The fluid droplets in the cornea scatter light rays, hence photophobia. The
dilatation of the eyeball is painful. Accordingly, *the presenting symptoms
are a constantly crying, fractious infant who keeps his eyes shut and his
head turned away from the light.* When the lids are gently opened by the
examiner's fingers, the enlarged, patchily opaque cornea with an enlarged
eyeball can be seen.
 Such patients should be referred within a few hours to an ophthalmic
surgeon for urgent operation.

Treatment

Treatment is surgical—goniotomy. Under general anaesthesia, a knife-needle is passed through peripheral cornea across the anterior chamber to incise the residual mesoderm in the angle. Only one quadrant can be treated at each operation, so repeat operations may be required to deal with a second, third or even fourth quadrant. An operation similar to trabeculectomy or trabeculotomy (*see* below) may be required in severe cases (e.g. with opaque corneae). The prognosis for eyes which have early operation is about 80–90% success. Parents should be warned of the risk to future children, viz. about 1 in 8 (these autosomal recessive genes have about 50% penetrance).

Angle-closure glaucoma

Mechanism

Patients who are destined to develop this disease, usually after the age of 50, are born with a shallow anterior chamber, which is associated with a small eyeball in overall dimensions, including a cornea with a small diameter (Fig 5.8). Their first-degree relatives tend to have the same

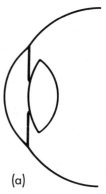 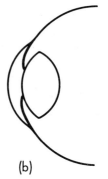 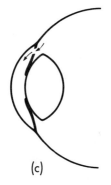

(a)   (b)   (c)

Fig 5.8 Anterior segments of eyeballs in cross-section. (a) An eye with open-angle glaucoma and a deep anterior chamber: the iris is all on one plane. (b) An eye predisposed to angle-closure glaucoma: the pupil is on a more anterior plane than the base of the iris and so the aqueous humour meets resistance at the pupil as it enters the anterior chamber, hence causing a ballooning forwards of the iris (iris bombé). The axial thickness of the lens is greater, surface curvatures of the lens are steeper and the corneal diameter is less than in open-angle glaucoma, all of which contribute to the shallow anterior chamber and the narrow angle. The lens goes on growing throughout life (in all eyes) so that the dangerously narrow angle eventually closes all round. (c) How a peripheral iridectomy or laser iridotomy will allow aqueous to pass through the hole in the iris, thereby eliminating the iris bombé and so making the angle of the anterior chamber much less narrow (though still narrower than in open-angle glaucoma because the contributing factors other than iris bombé still apply).

dimensions of eyeball and around 5% of them will also develop the disease in later life—i.e. there is a hereditary basis (exactly as in open-angle glaucoma, discussed below).

When the axial length of the eyeball is short, the rays of light passing through the pupil will tend to have a focal point behind the retina, when accommodation is relaxed—a state of hypermetropia (*see* Chapters 3 and 4). In an attempt to correct this refractive error, during development Nature makes the surfaces of the lens steeper so that the lens is axially thicker. Also the lens is more anteriorly placed in the eyeball. (The attribution to 'Nature' of a purpose is called 'teleological'. Although such rationalization would be of doubtful validity, given a belief in natural selection, it is frequently used as a basis for research hypotheses.)

The shallow anterior chamber is the resultant of all these factors (size, curvature and position of lens, short axial length of the eyeball and small diameter of cornea). *Accordingly the pupil is on a more anterior plane than the base of the iris*: this means that the angle of the anterior chamber is *abnormally narrow*. It also means that there is a resistance at the pupil margin to the free flow of aqueous humour into the anterior chamber, because the pupil area is more firmly applied to the lens than usual. In other words there is a higher than usual pressure in the aqueous behind the iris than there is in front. The iris therefore balloons forwards (iris bombé), rather like a spinnaker in the breeze, which makes *the angle of the anterior chamber even narrower*.

The extraordinary fact has already been mentioned that the lens in all eyes goes on increasing in size throughout life, with the laying down of layers of fibres as in an onion. Accordingly, in *all* eyes, the anterior chamber becomes shallower with increasing age (*see* Fig 8.1). In an eye with an already shallow anterior chamber, predisposing it to angle-closure glaucoma, the pupil will be pushed forwards increasingly, thereby narrowing the angle even more; the resistance to the flow of aqueous through the pupil will also increase so that the ballooning of the iris increases, and the angle of the anterior chamber will become still narrower: a diabolical situation.

Now, the angle of the anterior chamber is narrowest above and widest below, perhaps because the peripheral cornea is flatter above (*see* Plate 5.3). The peripheral iris in angle-closure glaucoma makes contact with, and blocks, the trabecular meshwork first of all at the 12 o'clock position. As the lens increases in size, the closure gradually proceeds downwards on the nasal and temporal side. When the pupil dilates slightly this contact-closure advances downwards; when it constricts (e.g. in the miosis which occurs in sleep) the contact-closure recedes upwards. When, say, around 50% of the angle is closed, subacute attacks of angle-closure glaucoma develop, usually in the early evening or in the darkness of the cinema when the pupil dilates slightly. The intraocular pressure rises within an hour or so, which produces discomfort or pain in the eye and multiple fine droplets of corneal oedema. These are responsible for the patient's sometimes seeing coloured rings round lights ('haloes') but this is not a very reliable symptom of angle-closure glaucoma*: the tiny droplets break up white light into its constituent colours as happens in a rainbow. Such attacks may occur for a few weeks or months on some or many evenings (*not* all) but eventually 'acute closed-angle glaucoma' occurs (*see* below) in about half of such cases.

Note on terminology
My usage of the term 'angle-closure' implies only *contact*-closure (reversible) between the peripheral iris and the trabecular meshwork. 'Closed-angle' implies *permanent* goniosynechia—i.e. irreversible closure of the meshwork by peripheral iris, probably with fibrosis as a late phenomenon.

In about one-third of cases, chronic closed-angle glaucoma evolves, with raised pressure, pathological cupping of the optic disc and field loss. This simulates chronic simple glaucoma (*see* below)—i.e. the presenting state is *not* acute closed-angle glaucoma.

Acute angle-closure (or closed-angle) glaucoma (see Plate 5.4)
About half the cases of *angle-closure glaucoma* present with an acute attack of *angle-closure (closed-angle) glaucoma* with or without a previous history of attacks of transient subacute glaucoma. The old name 'acute congestive glaucoma' is descriptive but was based on the erroneous belief that the cause was vascular instability. It results from complete closure of the whole angle of the anterior chamber—i.e. the ballooned peripheral iris closes the trabecular meshwork all round its full extent. That state has evolved from the progressive superior → inferior closure described above, the final total closure being quite sudden—and difficult to explain. Aqueous humour goes on being secreted into the eye but can no longer escape. The pressure rises very quickly to around 50 mmHg, causing severe pain, often with vomiting, redness of the conjunctiva, and multiple droplets of corneal oedema which make it rather difficult for the observer to see the iris and the vertically oval pupil. *The corneal oedema also reduces the patient's visual acuity*, which is a most important part of the diagnosis: the degree of impairment varies—usually 6/60 or less but it may be as good as 6/24 or 6/18. The patient usually presents with one eye affected for 24–48 hours; he should have pilocarpine (4% or 2% or 1%) once every five minutes instilled into the affected eye during urgent

---

* Early cataract is the commonest cause of haloes. They can also sometimes occur in open-angle glaucoma.

transit to an ophthalmic surgeon. *In this, as in many other eye diseases, the other eye is even more important than the affected eye*: the fellow eye has the same anatomical-mechanical predisposition as the affected eye and should have *prophylactically pilocarpine 0.5% or 1% every three hours until a peripheral iridectomy or laser iridotomy can be done*. Occasionally, bilateral acute angle-closure glaucoma occurs.

Early diagnosis or prevention may depend on the doctor's noticing a small eyeball with a small-diameter cornea. These may be easier to detect than the shallow anterior chamber; since that is due to the anterior position of the pupil, it may be made more obvious by shining a light from the temporal side on to the anterior segment of the eye and noting that the nasal half of the iris is in shadow. Do not use a mydriatic on such an eye—you may provoke acute angle-closure glaucoma.

Treatment

The ophthalmic surgeon will reduce the intraocular pressure with acetazolamide IM or IV and/or on intravenous drip of hypertonic mannitol (as is done by the neurosurgeon to reduce intracranial pressure). He may or may not wait for a few days, giving steroid eyedrops, until the hyperaemia settles down before doing an iridectomy (or laser iridotomy) or drainage operation. The iridectomy or laser iridotomy will eliminate the iris bombé. In the operation of (peripheral) iridectomy, under general or local anaesthesia, a conjunctival flap is mobilized in the 12 o'clock region as in drainage operations (*see* Fig 5.11). Then an incision at the limbus is made through the full thickness of the corneoscleral junction into the anterior chamber. The iris is elastic and its periphery will prolapse through this wound; the surgeon then excises a small piece and pushes the remainder of the iris back into the eyeball. The argon laser, however, is being increasingly used to make a peripheral iridotomy, which avoids the open operation, if the acute attack has been present for less than 24 hours.

Enough angle may thus be freed from fixed goniosynechiae to allow enough drainage of aqueous humour to reduce intraocular pressure to reasonably normal levels. If the 'acute attack' has been present for several days or more, an iridectomy alone will be inadequate because, say, 75% of the angle will be closed by permanent goniosynechiae; a drainage operation will then be required (*see* below).

About a week or so later, a prophylactic peripheral iridectomy or laser iridotomy will be done on the fellow eye—after gonioscopy to confirm that the angle is open, though it will almost invariably be dangerously narrow (*see* Plate 5.3). If the fellow eye has chronic closed-angle glaucoma, a drainage operation will be necessary (*see* Fig 5.11).

Subsequently, if it turns out that either peripheral iridectomy or drainage operation has been inadequate to maintain intraocular pressure below, say, 24 mmHg, additional long-term medical treatment will be required. The first choice will be timolol 0.25% or 0.5% once or twice daily because it has no effect on the pupil (*see* below). Pilocarpine unfortunately tends to produce 'posterior synechiae'—i.e. fibrous adhesions (NB not goniosynechiae)—between pupil and lens, because of the close contact between them and because aqueous no longer passes through the pupil; all of it will choose the line of least resistance through the iridectomy. A second operation—a drainage operation—is occasionally required (*see* below).

Open-angle (chronic simple) glaucoma

The cause of this disease is inadequacy of the mechanism by which aqueous humour passes through the endothelial layer of the trabecular meshwork. The exact biophysical basis is unknown. The defect has an important hereditary element since around 5% of first-degree relatives of patients also will have the disease when they reach the 50+ age group—exactly as in angle-closure glaucoma. On gonioscopy, the angle of the anterior chamber is, of course, open all round although it may be narrow.

At first, baseline intraocular pressure rises, and the normal diurnal variations increase: the approximate safety level of 24 mmHg is often transgressed. The patient practically never has pain or discomfort, and indeed considerable loss of peripheral field of vision may occur in one or both eyes before (s)he notices it.

The optic disc is the softest or most pressure-susceptible part of the whole eyeball. The corneoscleral envelope itself has very limited ability to expand or contract. The raised pressure pushes the optic disc backwards: at first the physiological cup enlarges and the surrounding disc tissue also becomes concave. As the months or years progress, the cup goes on enlarging. Unfortunately, the size of the cup in relation to the disc (cup to disc ratio, best measured in the vertical meridian) varies widely in normal eyes, like height, and is itself hereditary.

An eye with a vertical cup to disc (C/D) ratio of 0.5 or less has a very slight probability of having open-angle glaucoma. This probability rises with increasing C/D ratio until at 0.75 the probability is around 65% [1]. At any level, a difference in C/D ratio between the right and left eye of 0.2 or more (in practice any difference detectable ophthalmoscopically) increases the probability considerably.

The pattern of field loss (i.e. shape of the scotomata) is practically diagnostic of glaucoma, open-angle *and* chronic closed-angle, and is

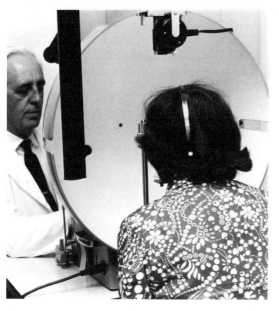

Fig 5.9 Field plotting on the Goldmann perimeter. The patient sits with her head supported on the chinrest, adjusted to site the left eye opposite the black fixation spot in the centre of the white bowl of the perimeter. The right eye is occluded. The patient looks at the black spot directly throughout the test with the left eye. A spot of light is projected at the periphery of the bowl and is moved gradually towards the centre: the patient signals as soon as the light is seen, and signals if it disappears anywhere en route to the centre of the bowl.

plotted in various ways (e.g. Goldmann perimeter—Fig 5.9). The mechanism of field loss is either through pressure on the blood supply of the appropriate sectors of the disc itself or direct mechanical pressure on the retinal nerve fibres as they pass over the edge of the disc. The first defect is usually an arcuate scotoma* passing from the blind spot up and over fixation—corresponding with the arching of the retinal nerve fibres (Fig 5.10). The next loss tends to be in the superonasal periphery, with a very characteristic 'nasal step'. Both of these progress, and an inferior arcuate scotoma is added, with inferonasal peripheral loss. Over a period of years, all peripheral field disappears, to leave, say, only 10 degrees of the central field; that island of vision is more slowly eroded to 5, 3, 2 degrees and finally the tiny residual islet is engulfed in the rising tide of blindness.

Early diagnosis is important because the patient may not notice field loss until late in the disease. Most cases are diagnosed incidentally when the patient attends the optician (optometrist) or ophthalmologist (oculist) for change of reading spectacles: routine ophthalmoscopy reveals pathological cupping, and tonometry may show a raised intraocular pressure.

Treatment

Open-angle glaucoma tends to be treated medically in contrast to angle-closure glaucoma which is treated surgically. The use of *pilocarpine*

* Scotoma = blind area.

Fig 5.10 Fields of vision of the right eye in glaucoma.
(a) The patient's right eye is fixating on the point of crossing of the vertical and horizontal lines. The peripheral extent of the field (white area) is normal—well beyond 40 degrees towards the nasal (left) side and well beyond 50 degrees towards the temporal (right) side. The broad inverted comma represents a blind area typical of glaucoma, the 'arcuate scotoma', extending from the blind spot on the horizontal meridian up and centrally to arch over fixation.

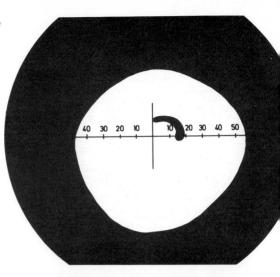

(b) This field shows more advanced glaucomatous loss—generalized constriction and extension of the arcuate scotoma to join an encroachment from the nasal periphery, limited below by the horizontal meridian ('nasal step').

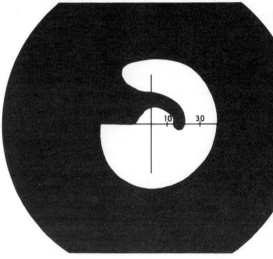

0.5%, 1%, 2% or 4% eyedrops three or four times daily is well established and effective. This parasympathomimetic drug stimulates directly the muscle cells of the ciliary body; when they contract, the mechanical pull on the trabecular meshwork causes—somehow—an increased outflow of aqueous humour: it 'opens up the outflow channels'. An unfortunate side effect in young people is an increase in accommodation which causes myopia. Another disadvantage for *all* patients is a small pupil (miosis) due to stimulation of the sphincter muscle of the pupil; that effect has no therapeutic value in open-angle

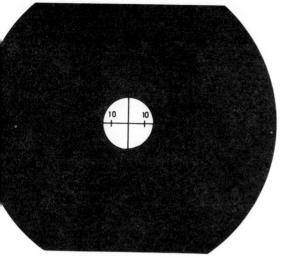

(c) This patient is suffering from advanced field loss: only 12–13 degrees of field around fixation remains. The next stage will be gradual erosion of this remaining island of vision until it is engulfed in the rising tide of blindness.

glaucoma (in contrast to its importance in angle-closure glaucoma—in which pilocarpine's effect on the ciliary muscle is a disadvantage!). An Ocusert* placed in the lower conjunctival fornix is effective for a week.

Another well established treatment is *adrenaline* 1% or 2% eyedrops twice daily. They reduce secretion of aqueous humour and increase outflow, by unknown mechanisms. An unfortunate side effect is stimulation of the dilator muscle of the pupil—unacceptable in angle-closure glaucoma but in open-angle glaucoma, in so far as it reduces the miosis of pilocarpine, it is an advantage. (Adrenaline and pilocarpine are often prescribed together in OAG.)

Rather surprisingly, given the effect of adrenaline, beta-adrenergic-blocking drugs topically (and systemically) reduce intraocular pressure. Timolol eyedrops 0.25% or 0.5% once or twice daily are in common use and are at least as efficacious as pilocarpine: they have no local side effects. This is a $beta_1$- and $beta_2$-blocker and acts by reducing secretion of aqueous humour. Absorption from the conjunctiva and nasal mucosa reduces pulse rate by around 10%; the drug should be avoided in patients with cardiac failure, bradycardia, asthma or bronchitis. Adrenaline's effect can be additive to timolol's unless and until beta-blockade in the eye is total, when adrenaline reduces timolol's effect.

Much less commonly used are phospholine iodide eyedrops 0.125% or 0.25% twice daily because it produces severe miosis and spasm of accommodation. It is a cholinesterase inhibitor, and systemic absorption

* An Ocusert (May & Baker) consists of a membrane of ethylene-vinyl acetate co-polymer with a matrix of alginic acid constituting a reservoir for pilocarpine.

reduces the level of the enzyme in the blood; that is dangerous only if succinylcholine is given as a relaxant for a general anaesthetic.

Forskolin eyedrops 1% have been shown to cause a fall in intraocular pressure, probably by reducing the volume of secreted aqueous humour [2]. It is a diterpene which acts directly on adenylate cyclase, without cell surface mediation, to increase intracellular levels of cyclic adenosine monophosphate (cAMP). Oral bromocriptine in eight human volunteers reduced intraocular pressure, possibly by stimulation of dopamine receptors [3].

Acetazolamide (Diamox) 250 mg twice daily by mouth, or 500 mg daily in enteric-coated capsules, reduces intraocular pressure by inhibiting carbonic anhydrase in the ciliary epithelium. Carbonic anhydrase is an enzyme which catalyses formation of H_2CO_3 from CO_2 and H_2O; H_2CO_3 normally combines with NaCl to produce sodium bicarbonate ($NaHCO_3$), which is an important constituent of aqueous humour. Presumably a reduction in the bicarbonate being secreted into aqueous humour reduces the water required to keep it in solution, hence reducing the total volume of fluid secreted by the ciliary epithelium, hence reducing intraocular pressure. Potassium lost in the urine should be replaced by supplements in the diet—600 mg potassium chloride daily in the middle of a meal, to avoid intestinal ulceration. Susceptible individuals may have pins-and-needles in the hands and feet. Renal stone formation is another small risk. Most ophthalmologists are reluctant to treat patients with acetazolamide on a long-term basis. Intramuscular or intravenous injection is often used to reduce intraocular pressure in acute angle-closure glaucoma.

Regular plotting of the fields of vision every 4–6 months is important in the monitoring of glaucoma patients. If maximum tolerable medical treatment fails to prevent continuing field loss, operation to increase the amount of aqueous outflow is necessary. Some surgeons prefer to operate earlier in the disease process.

Drainage operations
These increase the volume of fluid escaping from the eye into the subconjunctival space. From there, it probably seeps through the conjunctival epithelium to join the tears, rather than being absorbed into subconjunctival veins. The operation most commonly used at present is trabeculectomy (Fig 5.11c). Its original rationale was to eliminate a 3–4 mm length of trabecular meshwork, the site of abnormal resistance, and allow aqueous to go straight to the collector channels in the outer wall of Schlemm's canal, and possibly also to track along Schlemm's canal round the remainder of the limbus and obtain access to all the collector channels leaving the canal. However, we now believe that aqueous merely seeps through thinned sclera,

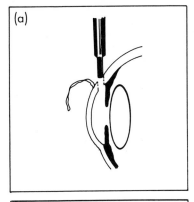

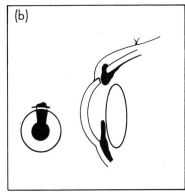

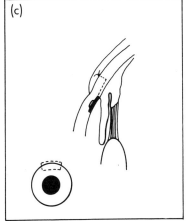

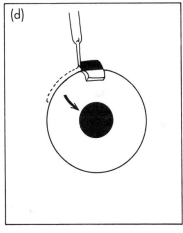

Fig 5.11 Drainage operations for open-angle (chronic simple) and chronic closed-angle glaucoma.

(a) Corneoscleral trephine is seldom done nowadays. A conjunctival flap is reflected forwards and a round hole 1.5 mm in diameter is drilled out of the corneoscleral junction. The conjunctival flap is sutured back into place, and aqueous from the anterior chamber flows into the subconjunctival space and seeps out through the conjunctiva into the tears.

(b) Iris inclusion also is unusual nowadays. A linear incision at the corneoscleral junction is about 4–5 mm long. A sector of iris is fashioned, remaining attached at its base, and placed in the linear incision to act as a wick and a wedge. Aqueous drains out as in the trephine.

(c) Trabeculectomy. After a conjunctival flap has been reflected forwards, a trapdoor of sclera is raised from behind forwards along the dotted lines, hinged anteriorly: the incision enters the canal of Schlemm along about 5 mm of its length. The trabecular meshwork plus some tissue in front of and behind it (dense black rectangle) is excised, and the scleral trapdoor and then the conjunctival flap are sutured into place. Aqueous probably seeps/trickles under the scleral trapdoor to reach the subconjunctival space rather than draining into the canal of Schlemm as was originally intended.

(d) Trabeculotomy is done in some centres. As in trabeculectomy, a scleral trapdoor hinged anteriorly is raised (under a conjunctival flap) to open the canal of Schlemm along 4 mm or so of its length. A probe (dotted line) is introduced along the canal: its handle is then rotated so that the probe moves in the direction of the arrow, into the anterior chamber, thereby breaking down the trabecular meshwork over almost one-quarter of its extent. The same manoeuvre is done on the other side of the trapdoor to add almost another quarter.

and round the edges of the trapdoor, to reach the subconjunctival space and thence to tears. (This operation was evolved from the ingenious trabeculotomy, now seldom used (Fig 5.11d). After the sclera flap has been raised, instead of excision of a length of meshwork as in trabeculectomy, a fine probe is inserted along Schlemm's canal on the nasal side for 3 hours of the clock and its handle turned to bring the probe into the anterior chamber, breaking down the trabecular meshwork in the process. The manoeuvre is repeated to the temporal side.)

Many patients attending glaucoma clinics will have had corneoscleral trephine operations (Fig 5.11a) and occasionally iris inclusions (Fig 5.11b). Nowadays, these operations are unusual.

There are important disadvantages in all such operations. There are the hazards of general or local anaesthesia; early mobilization minimizes some of these. Haemorrhage or infection at operation, or immediately afterwards, are uncommon. Any perforating injury—including drainage operation—will tend to produce cataract in the longer term even if the lens capsule has not been directly injured by instruments at operation (the slightest trauma to the lens capsule will usually cause total cataract within a few days). Glaucoma itself, and pilocarpine eyedrops also, are factors which predispose to cataract. In the case of corneoscleral trephine, if not trabeculectomy (Fig 5.11), only a thin layer of conjunctiva separates the intraocular contents from the outside, so conjunctivitis is very dangerous: organisms may easily pass into the eyeball and within days produce a tragic panophthalmitis. Sympathetic ophthalmitis is a rare complication.

Glaucoma complicating other pathological processes

'Secondary' is a more justifiable name to apply to this group of glaucomas than is the term 'primary' applied to open-angle and angle-closure glaucoma.

Around 5% of cases of *iridocyclitis* are complicated by a raised intraocular pressure, because the trabecular meshwork becomes clogged or silted up by white cells and by inflammatory exudate released by the iris and ciliary body into the aqueous humour. Such cases may well have a pre-existing predisposition to open-angle or angle-closure glaucoma.

Iridocyclitis may rarely produce glaucoma by another mechanism. If the whole pupil becomes bound down to the anterior surface of the lens (total posterior synechiae), no aqueous humour can reach the anterior chamber: it accumulates quickly behind the iris which balloons *very markedly* forwards (much more so than in angle-closure glaucoma) so that its periphery blocks the whole trabecular meshwork to cause a very high rise of pressure. This possible danger explains why we treat iridocyclitis vigorously with atropine and phenylephrine 10% eyedrops and steroids to minimize posterior synechiae.

Steroid eyedrops for a few weeks will produce insidious steroid glaucoma in 10–20% of the population. It has the same characteristics as open-angle glaucoma: indeed a (hereditary) predisposition to that disease is probably a prerequisite for a dangerous rise in pressure from topical steroids. However, steroid-induced glaucoma will occur in eyes which might well otherwise never develop overt glaucoma. Withdrawal of the steroid eyedrops usually allows the glaucoma to resolve, but such patients are worth regular annual checks in their future. Systemic steroids have a very much smaller effect on intraocular pressure, presumably because their concentration at the trabecular meshwork is much lower. Many cases are on record in which steroid eyedrops prescribed for 'chronic conjunctivitis' have tragically produced blindness.

All ophthalmologists issue regular warnings to general practitioners to avoid topical steroids unless prescribed *and* monitored by a specialist. (There is also a risk of aggravation of dendritic (herpetic) corneal ulcers if steroids are given to a 'red eye' without an accurate diagnosis.)

Neovascular glaucoma represents a nice piece of experimental work which Nature performs for us—unfortunately. If a retina becomes ischaemic from central retinal vein occlusion or diabetic retinopathy, some chemical with the property of stimulating capillary new growth diffuses outwards, hence new vessel formation in the retina and in the optic disc: some diffuses through the vitreous into aqueous humour and stimulates new vessel formation in the iris *and in the angle of the anterior chamber.* Accordingly, the trabecular meshwork is covered by a thin fibrovascular sheet to produce a particularly intractable glaucoma. The chemical nature of this rather hypothetical but very interesting substance has not yet been established.

Other causes of 'secondary' glaucoma are much more rare; for example, a swollen ('intumescent') cataractous lens may push the peripheral iris against the whole of the trabecular meshwork. Concussion of the eyeball may dislocate the lens forwards with the same result. A malignant melanoma from the ciliary body might infiltrate the whole angle and trabecular meshwork.

Prevention and early diagnosis

Few ophthalmologists advocate screening of the general population to detect unsuspected glaucoma; however, this is already being done in so far as almost all patients over 45 years are seen every few years by an optician or ophthalmologist for reading spectacles. At these consultations, the optic discs will be inspected and in many cases tonometry will be done.

A good case can be made for seeking out and examining first-degree relatives of glaucoma patients over the age of 50. The usual problems in any screening programme apply—expense in administration, false-positive and false-negative results, relatives already under care, etc.

References

1 Gloster J (1980) The relationship of optic disc and visual field changes in glaucoma. In *Research and Clinical Forums*, vol. 2, pp. 137–46. Ed. Pitts Crick, R.
2 Caprioli J and Sears M (1983) Forskolin lowers intraocular pressure in rabbits, monkeys and man. *Lancet* **1**, 958–60
3 Mekki Q A, Hassan S M and Turner P (1983) Bromocriptine lowers intra-ocular pressure without affecting blood pressure. *Lancet* **1**, 1250–1

6 The Red Eye

C I Phillips

The differential diagnosis of the red eye as a presenting symptom is very important because the causes range from the relatively trivial foreign body in the lower conjunctival fornix to acute closed-angle glaucoma and iridocyclitis. The pivot of the diagnosis is the visual acuity. If reduced, the condition is serious; if normal, it may not be. The points to look for are summarized in Table 6.1.

Foreign bodies are considered in Chapter 11, under 'Trauma'. The history usually gives the diagnosis.

Acute closed-angle glaucoma is described in Chapter 5.

Acute bacterial conjunctivitis

Infection with a pyogenic organism such as staphylococcus or pneumococcus is invariably bilateral, but sometimes not quite simultaneous in onset within the first day. Visual acuity is normal, and any age group may be affected. There is no mistaking the mucopus on the lid margins which cause the eyelids to stick together after a night's sleep. The conjunctiva covering the eyeballs is diffusely red, and this extends equally into the upper and lower fornices on both sides. Both eyes water profusely.

Eyedrops and oculentum* of a broad spectrum antibiotic are the basis of treatment. The patient lies on a couch or bed with head low. The therapist lifts each upper lid in turn to dribble one or two drops underneath it into the upper fornix where inaccessible organisms may otherwise lurk. For the first five minutes, this is done every minute; for the remainder of an hour, it is repeated once every five minutes. Thus, a

---

* An ointment for use in the conjunctival sac.

Symptoms	Acute angle-closure (closed-angle) glaucoma	Acute iridocyclitis	Conjunctivitis — Acute bacterial	Conjunctivitis — Acute adenovirus	Keratitis and corneal ulcers
Previous history	Episodes of blurring, pain or haloes for an hour or two in some early evenings	Any previous attack protracted for weeks	Possible	Sometimes	Previous attacks frequent in viral types. Foreign body or other injury
Pain	Severe, radiating to forehead, with vomiting	Moderate, more localized to eye. Dull	Gritty, especially on blinking	Gritty, especially on blinking	Moderate to severe. Sharp on blinking
Photophobia	Slight	Moderate	Slight	Slight/moderate	Marked
Secretion	Watery	Watery	(Muco-)purulent: heavy	Watery	Watery ++
Visual acuity	Bad	Poor or slightly reduced	Normal	Normal	Poor to bad
Onset	Within 2–3 hours	Gradual (1–2 days)	Within 1–2 days	Several days	Gradual (1–2 days)
Systemic symptoms	Prostration and vomiting because of pain	Malaise or none	None	None	None
Bilateral?	Unilateral usually	Unilateral usually	Invariably bilateral	Unilateral or bilateral	Unilateral usually
Age	Usually 50+	Usually 15–25	Any, but usually in children	Any, but usually up to 25	Any

| | Acute angle-closure (closed-angle) glaucoma | Acute iridocyclitis | Conjunctivitis | | Keratitis and corneal ulcers |
			Acute bacterial	Acute adenovirus	
Signs					
Hyperaemia	Circumcorneal purple ± diffuse conjunctival	Circumcorneal purple ± diffuse conjunctival	Conjunctival, severe and diffuse. Brick red	Conjunctival, mild. Often restricted to sector next to limbus	Circumcorneal purple
Pupil	Dilated. Oval	Contracted. Irregular	Normal	Normal	Usually contracted, if visible.
Pupil light reflex	Absent or reduced	Reduced or absent	Normal	Normal	Reduced or absent
Cornea	Epithelial oedema (fogging view of iris)	(Keratic) precipitates	Clear and sparkling	Clear and sparkling; sector may show punctate stains/infiltrates on slit-lamp microscopy	Grey area or stains with fluorescein/rose bengal
Anterior chamber	Shallow (NB see fellow eye)	Exudate (flare; cells). Often deep. Sometimes hypopyon	Normal	Normal	As in iridocyclitis. Often hypopyon
Iris	Oedematous and hyperaemic	Often hyperaemic and 'muddy'	Normal	Normal	Usually hyperaemic
Tension	Very high	High, normal or low	Normal	Normal	Usually normal to low
Tenderness	Marked	Moderate to marked	Slight	Slight	Marked
Other points	Parent or sibling may have had emergency eye operation	Ankylosing spondylitis in males	Epidemic in school or family?	Epidemic at school or work?	History of injury usually

Table 6.1 Differential diagnosis: the red eye

loading dose of antibiotic can be achieved in spite of the tendency for the excessive tear production to wash the drug away. For the remainder of the day, drops are instilled every hour. Just before the patient goes to bed, oculentum is squirted instead into the lower fornices: this maintains action during the night better than drops and also prevents drying of crusts of pus on the lid margin. No pad should be put over the eye, even at night—free drainage of pus must be allowed. For 4 or 5 days, drops should be used every 3–4 hours, more conveniently into the lower fornix now that the acute stage is past; oculentum at night should continue. Depending on individual circumstances, treatment should continue at least until the seventh or eighth day.

Epidemic spread must be prevented, especially in institutions. The patient and therapist must 'scrub up' before and after touching or treating the eyes. Cotton wool swabs, preferably sterile, soaked in warm saline (1 teaspoonful salt to 1 pint water), should be used to wipe away crusts and mucopus mechanically from the lid margins—and destroyed immediately after use. The patient should have his own towel and pillow, to be thoroughly laundered when he has recovered. Antibiotic drops are usually supplied in drop bottles: great care must be taken, of course, not to contaminate the tip of the dropper on the lids or lashes because it is easy then to contaminate the whole bottle of drops and so keep on reinfecting the eyes. Other individuals must not share the use of the bottle!

If a newborn child is affected by severe conjunctivitis ('ophthalmia neonatorum') *gonococcal conjunctivitis* should be suspected, and cultures and smears taken. Vulvovaginitis with the same organism in a female child may also be present. The mother's birth canal and the father's genitalia should be investigated to establish the source. The effectiveness of intensive penicillin eyedrops may be reduced because of epiphora and production of pus, so daily intramuscular crystalline penicillin 50 000–100 000 units are advisable. For beta-lactamase-producing gonococci, cefuroxin or spectinomycin systemically may be necessary. The cornea should be inspected daily to exclude ulceration.

Another cause of conjunctivitis with or without vulvovaginitis in the newborn is the *Chlamydia trachomatis*, which is also a major cause of 'non-specific urethritis' in the adult, and less commonly anoproctitis, presumably because of similarities between the conjunctival mucosa and the genitourinary mucosa. The clinical presentation includes acute mucopurulent discharge, and the diagnosis can be missed because of coexisting gonorrhoea. Serotypes D to K affect mainly the genitourinary mucosa but quite often the conjunctiva; serotypes A to C cause trachoma (*see* Chapter 15) but seldom infect the genital mucosa.

Adenovirus conjunctivitis

This is more properly keratoconjunctivitis because the corneal epithelium is involved, is usually unilateral and mild with slight watering, and some redness. Often the hyperaemia is maximal in one sector, usually inferotemporally, and extends 3–5 mm from the limbus. The related sector of cornea will usually show small infiltrates or spots of epithelial damage on slit-lamp microscopy. The pre-auricular lymph node will be enlarged and tender in severe cases. Visual acuity is usually normal. Although the disease is self-limiting and antibiotics are almost powerless, they are usually prescribed as for bacterial conjunctivitis: at least they prevent secondary infection and the oculentum will reduce soreness in the eye which is due to mechanical rubbing of uneven tender surfaces on blinking. Again, epidemic spread should be prevented as for bacterial conjunctivitis.

Herpetic keratitis (dendritic ulcer)

The virus of herpes simplex causes a typical 'dendritic' corneal ulcer, with an associated conjunctivitis and epiphora *without* mucopurulent discharge (*see* Plate 6.1). Surprisingly, it is almost always unilateral. Pain, especially on blinking, and photophobia are usually obvious. The ulcer may be small and not easily visible even with focal illumination and magnification: fluorescein or rose-bengal eyedrops will stain the damaged epithelium along the edge of the ulcer to show its diagnostic pattern—it branches into rootlets (hence 'dendritic') along its length and at its ends (*see* Plate 6.1). Visual acuity may be considerably reduced if the ulcer is in the centre of the cornea but only slightly reduced if the ulcer is peripheral.

Treatment is traditionally by carbolization or iodization or by mechanical débridement of the infected area of corneal epithelium; idoxuridine or cytarabine (cytosine arabinoside) or vidarabine (adenine arabinoside) or acyclovir eyedrops hourly for a few days, however, are often successful. Recurrences are not uncommon, so these treatments may have to be repeated. A serious complication occurs occasionally when the organism spreads deeply into the central cornea, with grey–white opacification due to oedema and inflammatory infiltrates (later vascularization from the limbus), possibly with an allergic element in addition. '*Disciform keratitis*' describes this central opaque area which typically has fairly clear surrounding cornea. Ophthalmologists regularly see patients with a unilateral red eye in which the diagnosis of dendritic ulcer has been missed and which have been treated with topical steroids with or without antibiotics: the result is reduction of symptoms but disastrous spread of the infection, often deeply. Any red eye which *might* have a dendritic ulcer *must not* be treated with steroids.

Corneal ulcers

These are associated with a variety of organisms, other than herpes simplex virus, the infection usually being initiated by injury to the corneal epithelium. Pyogenic organisms are commonest, and produce a grey–white slough at the site of the lesion (*see* Plate 11.1a). The toxic products from the ulcer diffuse into the anterior chamber (as well as towards the limbus) and excite an inflammatory response from the blood vessels of the iris; the pus cells gravitate to the bottom of the anterior chamber and show the characteristic horizontal line of a 'hypopyon' (*see* Plate 11.1b). Pain and epiphora are usually severe. An infection by fungi, usually following an agriculture injury, evolves more slowly in the cornea, usually without a hypopyon: branching hyphae from the ulcer may be seen with the slit-lamp microscope.

Treatment is by a broad spectrum antibiotic—usually by subconjunctival injection initially, until the organism and its sensitivities have been established by smears and cultures. Pimaricin drops intensively are a useful first approximation for fungus infections.

Iridocyclitis

This is an uncommon cause of a red watering eye but the diagnosis must always be considered because serious consequences can result from missing it (*see* Plate 6.2). Inflammation in the iris and ciliary body 'irritates' the sphincter muscle of the pupil which becomes small (and reacts poorly, if at all, for near and on accommodation) and also irritates the ciliary muscle, which may account for the constant dull ache which is usually present. Visual acuity is slightly (or markedly) reduced by the slight (or severe) inflammatory exudate in the anterior chamber, in the pupil and in the anterior vitreous. The reactive hyperaemia in the anterior uveal tract (iris and ciliary body) also affects the related blood vessels of the anterior sclera, especially around the limbus, to produce the characteristic circumcorneal red–blue blush, but diffuse conjunctival hyperaemia is often also present. Some epiphora is common but *there is no mucopurulent exudate in the conjunctival sac, of course*. This disease is usually unilateral, only occasionally bilateral. When severe, the intraocular pressure may be high.

Agglutination and sedimentation of the rather few white cells in the inflammatory exudate in the anterior chamber produce deposits on the back of the lower cornea—'keratic precipitates' (KP)—and a careful search for these should be made to establish the diagnosis. Especially in early or mild cases, a slit-lamp microscope may be needed to make the diagnosis.

'Posterior synechiae' are almost diagnostic of iridocyclitis: the pupil is bound down to the underlying lens by sticky inflammatory exudate. Attempted dilatation of the pupil with a mydriatic will show areas of the pupil to be stuck down and other areas successfully dilating, producing an irregular or festooned pupil. The risk of the disaster of total posterior synechiae, grossly ballooned iris and severe glaucoma (*see* 'secondary glaucoma' in Chapter 5) is high unless vigorous treatment with mydriatics (atropine *and* phenylephrine) and, usually, steroids is given.

No systemic cause for iridocyclitis can usually be identified. However, it is a well-known recurrent complication of ankylosing spondylitis: a history of low backache would be expected in that condition. A low-grade chronic form is associated with sarcoidosis. Occasionally it may be caused by tuberculosis or syphilis.

Other causes of 'sore eyes'

Allergic conjunctivitis

Allergic conjunctivitis is usually easy to diagnose because it is associated with other evidence such as 'hay fever', asthma, etc. Treatment is by antazoline (Antistin-Privine) eyedrops. A particular variety, *vernal* (or *spring*) *catarrh*, also usually seasonal, shows multiple 'cobblestones' (each 1–3 mm in diameter) of the tarsal conjunctiva when the upper lid is everted: if specific topical treatment with cromoglycate fails, steroid eyedrops usually control the condition—but steroid glaucoma is a definite risk, to be excluded by tonometry and other ophthalmic supervision.

Senile (or spastic) entropion

Senile entropion of the lower lid in an elderly person will produce a red sore eye which is usually surprisingly mild, because it tends to be intermittent at first. A small plastic operation is effective.

Trichiasis

Even one or two distorted eyelashes rubbing on conjunctiva or cornea may produce a feeling of a foreign body: previous injury or localized inflammation may be the cause. Electrolysis under local anaesthesia is the usual treatment.

Rosacea

Rosacea of the skin of the face is often associated with a recurrent low-grade degenerative inflammatory reaction of the conjunctiva and superficial cornea (with characteristic peripheral opacification and vascularization visible with the slit-lamp microscope). A six-week course of oxytetracycline by mouth (repeated occasionally if necessary) is surprisingly effective treatment. Topical steroids will also control symptoms but the risk of producing glaucoma is about 10–20%.

Sjögren's syndrome

This is an association of 'dry' eyes and a dry mouth with rheumatoid arthritis, not necessarily severe (*see* Chapter 14). There is hyposecretion of tears (and saliva) with stringy mucous in the lower fornix, and characteristic short ribbons of epithelial débris encased in mucus attached to cornea. The diagnosis is confirmed by Schirmer's test: a short narrow strip of sterile filter paper, 'hooked' into the lower lid, is wetted for a subnormal distance (usually less than 5 mm) at the end of a standard five minutes.

Watering eye or eyes without redness

This condition tends to occur in the early weeks or months of life or in the elderly (*see* Chapter 14). In both cases, the cause usually is a blockage of the nasolacrimal duct. When it is due to a congenital blockage which fails to resolve by the age of 6–9 months, a probe passed down the duct via the lacrimal punctum under general anaesthesia usually cures the condition. If epiphora in the elderly is troublesome, a dacryocystorhinostomy has a good success rate: flaps of lacrimal sac are stitched to matching flaps of nasal mucosa after removal of the thin lacrimal bone which separates the two. Blockage may exist at other sites, especially the junction of common canaliculus and sac: surgical intervention in that area is less successful.

Plate 1.1 Diagram of partly cut away forebrain vesicle of early embryo. An outpouching, the optic vesicle, has already developed an indentation on its ventral surface (*see also* Plate 1.2). The surface ectoderm, the future skin, hugs the lateral extremity of the optic vesicle (*see* Plate 1.3).

After Mann, Ida. *The Development of the Human Eye*. London: British Medical Association, 1964. *Reproduced by kind permission of author and publisher.*

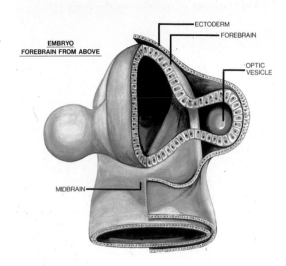

Plate 1.2 The ventral surface of the optic vesicle has become indented, and the development of the optic cup is well established. The fetal or ocular or choroidal fissure (i.e. the slit remaining between the edges of the indented area) later closes except for the two ends. The smaller gap becomes the optic disc. The larger gap at the other end of the fetal fissure is surrounded by the peripheral edge of the future retina.

After Mann, Ida. *The Development of the Human Eye*. London: British Medical Association, 1964. *Reproduced by kind permission of author and publisher.*

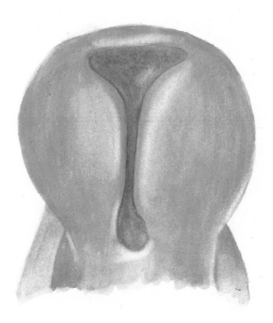

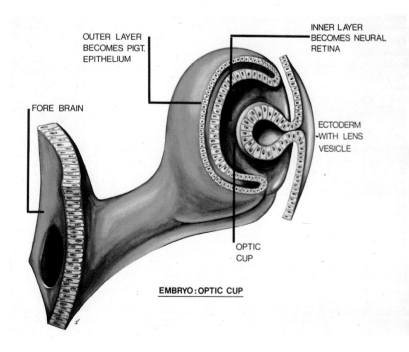

OUTER LAYER
BECOMES PIGT.
EPITHELIUM

INNER LAYER
BECOMES NEURAL
RETINA

FORE BRAIN

OPTIC
CUP

ECTODERM
WITH LENS
VESICLE

OPTIC
CUP

EMBRYO : OPTIC CUP

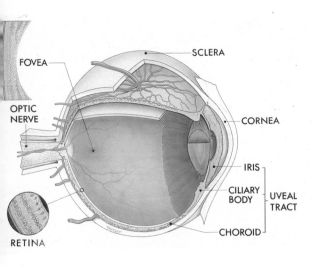

FOVEA

OPTIC
NERVE

RETINA

SCLERA

CORNEA

IRIS

CILIARY
BODY

CHOROID

UVEAL
TRACT

Plate 1.3 Diagram of the optic cup. The outer layer will remain single-celled to become the pigment epithelium of the adult retina, with Bruch's membrane outside it. The inner layer will form the remainder—i.e. the main part of the multilayered retina. Stimulated by the optic vesicle and cup, the adjacent surface ectoderm sends a hollow vesicle inwards, towards the cavity of the developing eyeball; it will form the lens of the eyeball, occupying a plane just anterior to the extreme edge of the retina. The bridge of tissue between the forebrain and optic vesicle will become the optic nerve.

Plate 1.4 Exploded diagram to show the anatomy of the eyeball.

Plate 5.1 Solid section of anterior segment of eyeball. Part of the dome of the cornea (anterior) is above in the painting. Aqueous humour in the anterior chamber drains into the canal of Schlemm through the trabecular meshwork. It is secreted by the epithelium covering the finger-like ciliary processes of the ciliary body; the processes also give origin to some of the suspensory ligament of the lens, and most of the ciliary body consists of ciliary muscle. It flows slowly through the suspensory ligament, round the lens and through the pupil to reach the anterior chamber.

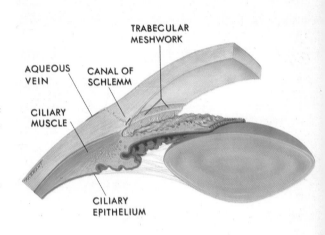

TRABECULAR MESHWORK

AQUEOUS VEIN

CANAL OF SCHLEMM

CILIARY MUSCLE

CILIARY EPITHELIUM

Plate 5.2 Applanation tonometry. Observer's view through the eyepieces of the slit-lamp microscope (see also Figs 5.1 and 5.2). Fluorescein eye drops have been instilled (after topical anaesthetic drops) so that the edge of the flattened area of cornea will show up as a yellow-green ring—there is a meniscus, wedge-shaped in cross-section, of fluorescein-stained tears surrounding the flattened area of cornea which has been cleared of tears. A doubling device in the prism converts the ring of meniscus round the flattened area into two half-rings to make it easy for the observer to judge the end-point. The central section of the painting shows this end-point when the force applied to the tonometer is enough to clear the standard area of cornea. The top section shows an underestimate of the end-point and the lowest section shows an overestimate.

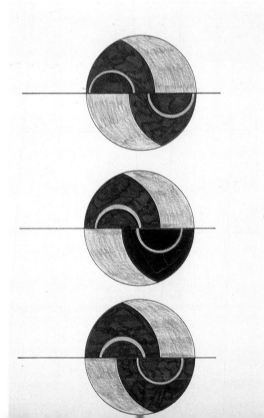

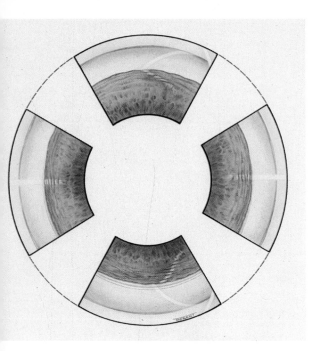

Plate 5.3 The angle of the anterior chamber in an eye progressing through the subclinical stage of angle-closure glaucoma. Superiorly, the base of the iris has occluded the trabecular meshwork; inferiorly, the angle is just open, allowing access of aqueous humour to the meshwork. In the 5–7 o'clock sector the trabecular meshwork can be identified just beyond the periphery of the iris as the inner (i.e. nearer the iris), broader of two lines running parallel with the iris's base. The transition between closed and open angle occurs at about 9 and 3 o'clock.

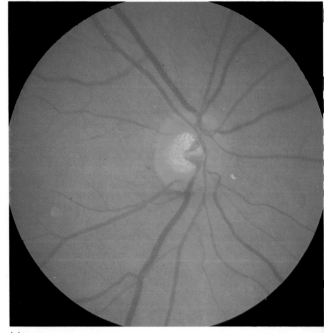

(a)

Plate 5.4 Acute closed-angle glaucoma (previously called acute congestive glaucoma). The predisposed angle (Plate 5.3) has completely closed because of gradual increase in axial thickness of lens with increasing ballooning of iris. The intraocular pressure has risen suddenly within half an hour or so, to produce a stony hard eyeball with severe pain, often vomiting, *poor visual acuity* (usually worse than 6/24), a vertically oval semi-dilated pupil and a 'steamy' cornea (with multiple droplets of oedema).

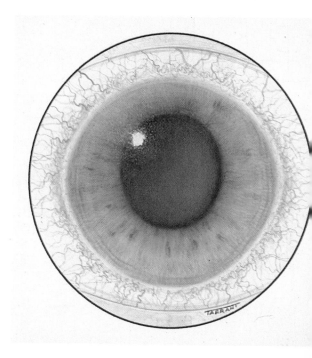

Plate 5.5 (a) and (b) The *right* optic disc (a) has a vertical cup-to-disc (C/D) ratio of about 0.75—i.e. very probably pathological. Do not mistake the edge of the circumpupillary halo (due to sclera seen through transparent retina, choroid being absent) for the edge of the disc. Early glaucomatous field loss is present and ocular tension is 22 mmHg. The *left* disc's vertical C/D ratio is about 0.66 (b). The arc of pigmentation on the temporal side is a common physiological finding. No glaucomatous field loss is present but ocular tension is also 22 mmHg. Note that the inequality between right and left C/D ratios is an important criterion for diagnosis of pathological cupping.

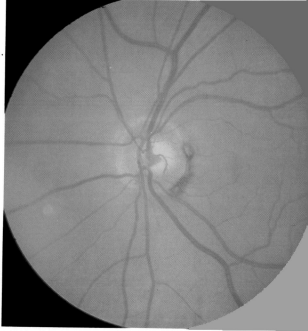

(b)

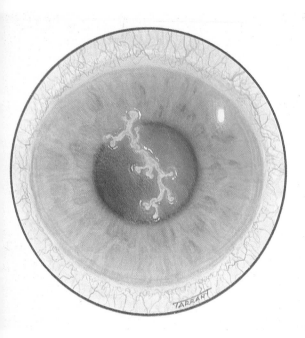

Plate 6.1 Large dendritic corneal ulcer stained by fluorescein. The excess has been washed off with two or three drops of saline eyedrops.

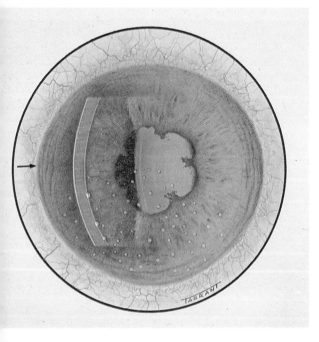

Plate 6.2 Iridocyclitis. Atropine 1% and phenylephrine 10% have dilated some parts of the pupil, leaving five or six points where the pupil is stuck to the anterior lens capsule—'posterior synechiae'. The beam of the slit-lamp microscope, coming from the observer's left, traverses the cornea and shows that the white keratic precipitates (KP) are scattered over the *endothelial* (posterior) surface of the lower half of the cornea. These KP are aggregated clumps of white cells in the aqueous humour (seen as glistening dots in the beam of the slit-lamp as it traverses the anterior chamber) which have gravitated downwards. 'Flare' is present, shown by the visibility of the slit beam as it traverses the normally optically empty anterior chamber; subcellular inflammatory exudate in the aqueous humour scatters some light in the beam.

Plate 7.1 Central retinal artery occlusion. Note the thin retinal arterioles. The main evidence of infarction is in the thickest area of retina, hazy white, surrounding the fovea which is the red dot, two and a half disc diameters temporal to the disc. The fovea, being thin, is transparent and allows the red highly vascular normal choroid to show through: cherry red spot.

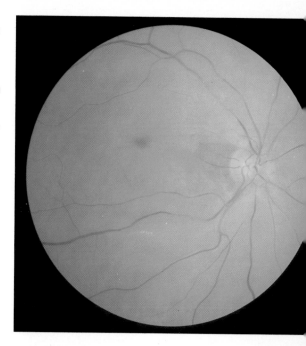

Plate 7.2 Central retinal vein occlusion. Splashes of haemorrhage radiate from the oedematous optic disc, with scattered exudates. Haemorrhages extend outwards into peripheral retina (not seen in the picture). In contrast, papilloedema due to raised intracranial pressure is strictly localized to the disc area (with very few haemorrhages in the early stages).

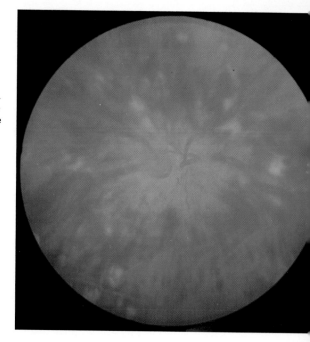

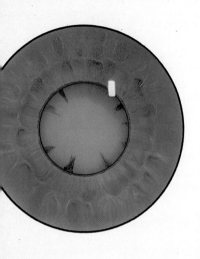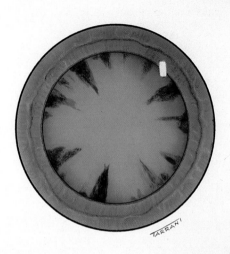

8.1 ▲

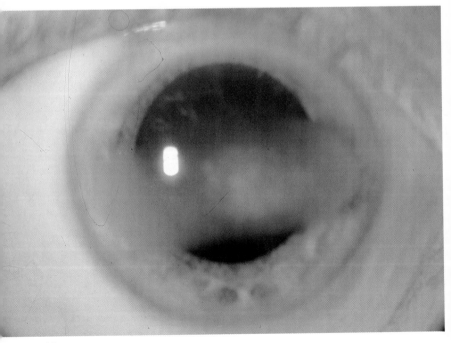

8.2 ▲

88 Basic Clinical Ophthalmology

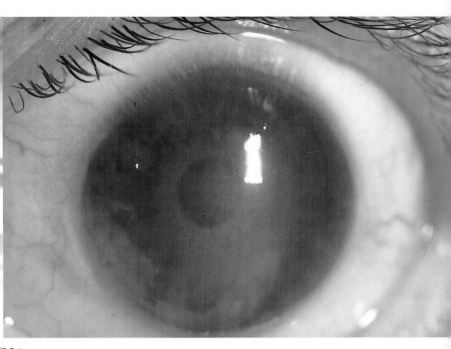

8.3 ▲

Plate 8.1 Cuneiform lens opacities (more visible through dilated pupil) seen as black wedge-shaped silhouettes on a red background. (*See* Chapter 2.)

Plate 8.2 Band-shaped keratopathy in an elderly patient with no history of systemic or other ocular disease.

Plate 8.3 Lattice degeneration of the cornea producing a central diffuse opacity and a reduction of the visual acuity to 6/24.

Plate 8.4 A slit-lamp photograph of a successful penetrating keratoplasty. There is a continuous monofilament nylon suture in position.

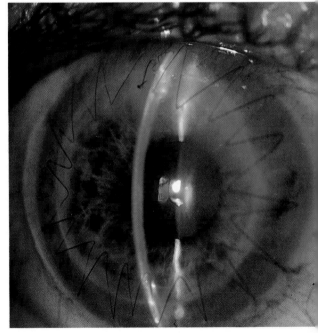

8.4 ▲

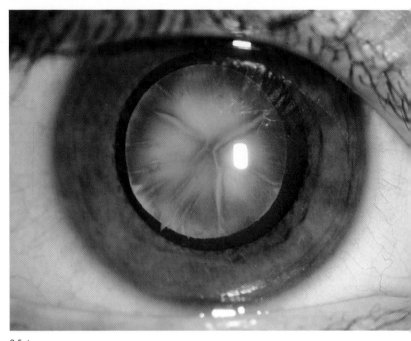

8.5 ▲

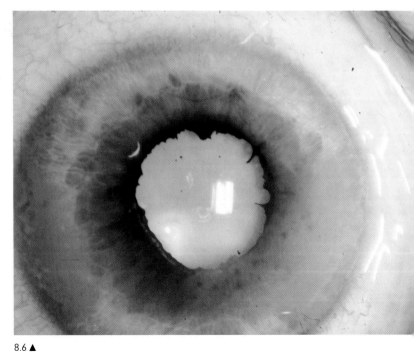

8.6 ▲

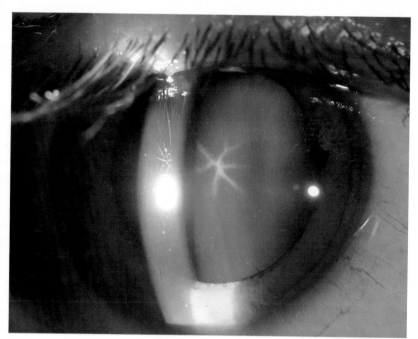

8.7 ▲

Plate 8.5 A congenital lamellar cataract in a 10-year-old child.

Plate 8.6 A mature cataract in a patient with a history of recurrent uveitis and Still's disease. Early band-shaped keratopathy can be seen.

Plate 8.7 Anterior sutural lens opacities occurring in a patient treated with long-term chlorpromazine.

Plate 8.8 Macular degeneration occurring in an elderly patient. This particular, rather unusual, example is known as central choroidal sclerosis.

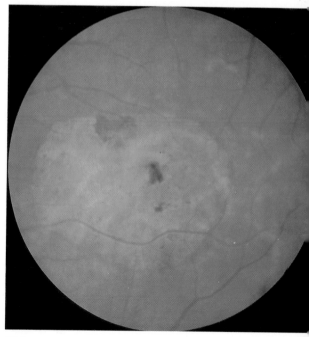

8.8 ▲

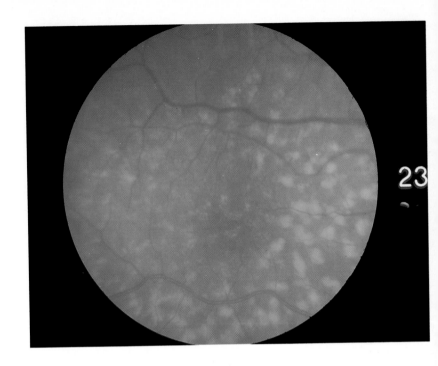

23

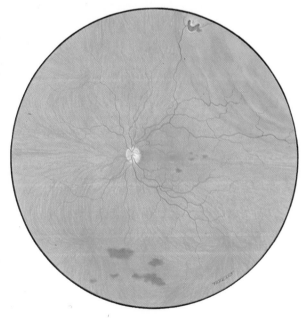

Plate 8.9 Multiple colloid bodies around the posterior pole. They are seen in association with macular degeneration in the elderly.

Plate 8.10 Cavitation and collapse of the vitreous (with some slowly accumulating vitreous 'floaters') has resulted in detachment of vitreous from the retina—always from behind forwards. It has pulled on a vitreoretinal adhesion to produce an arrowhead tear (pointing towards the disc, of course) plus a *very sudden* small 'snowstorm' of floaters due to tearing of a retinal capillary, with a small vitreous haemorrhage of which traces can still be seen. Fluid has seeped through the retinal hole to cause a *progressive retinal detachment.*

(See **Plate 8.11** *opposite*)

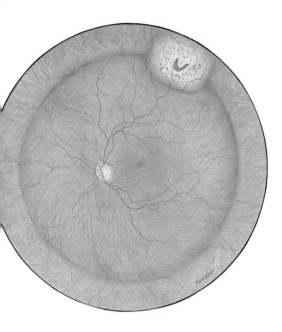

Plate 8.11 The surgeon applies a cryoprobe to the surface of the sclera to produce an area of 'sticky' mild choroiditis in the region of the retinal hole. He sutures a silicone plomb to the scleral surface in the same area, to drive the wall of the eyeball inwards after he has released subretinal fluid through a sclerotomy wound. An encircling silicone band raises a ridge all round the peripheral retina which relieves the traction of fine vitreous bands and holds the plomb in place, thereby preventing recurrences. (*See* **Plate 8.10** *opposite*, also **Fig 8.4**.)

Plate 10.1 Left posterior fundus of patient with long-standing essential hypertension. The retinal arteries show moderate sclerosis, and arteriovenous crossing changes are pronounced superior to left optic disc. The macular branch of the superotemporal artery is irregular and attenuated, and occasional microaneurysms, dilated capillaries and nerve fibre haemorrhage are present.

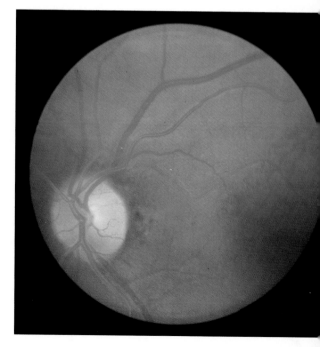

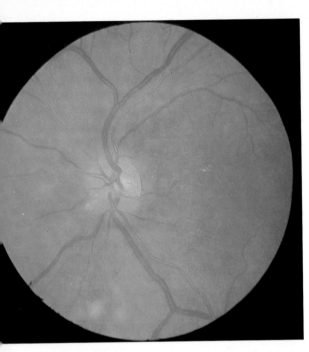

Plate 10.2 Left posterior fundus of patient with severe essential hypertension. The arteries are sclerosed, irregular and attenuated. There is moderate retinopathy (hard exudates, microaneurysms and haemorrhages) and multiple foci of inner retinal ischaemia (cotton wool spots).

Plate 10.3 Left posterior fundus of patient with severe accelerated hypertension. There is widespread inner retinal ischaemia with conglomerations of cotton wool spots and intraretinal haemorrhages. The retinal arterioles are markedly constricted and the superior optic disc is swollen.

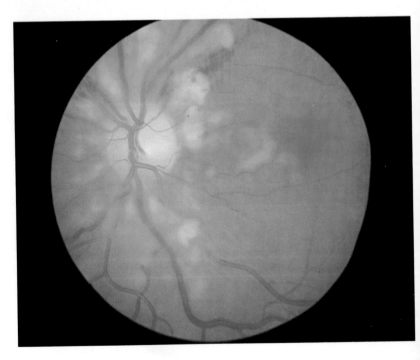

Plate 10.4 Left posterior fundus of patient with severe accelerated hypertension. The retinal arterioles are severely constricted and in some areas occluded (nasal field and superior to disc). A superotemporal vein is occluded at an arteriovenous crossing and fronds of new vessels have developed at the optic disc in response to the widespread inner retinal ischaemia.

Plate 10.5 Left superotemporal fundus of patient with long-standing severe hypertension and carotid artery disease. The arteries are irregular and attenuated, and occasional intraretinal haemorrhages and cotton wool spots are present. Cholesterol emboli are impacted along the course of the superonasal and superotemporal arteries.

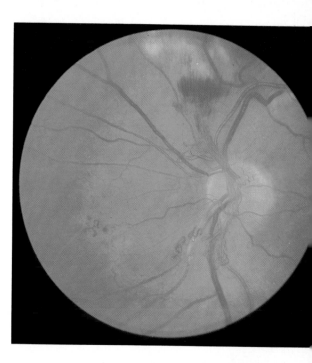

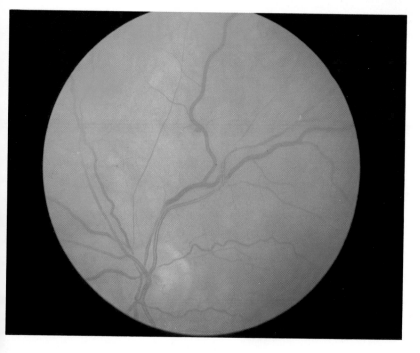

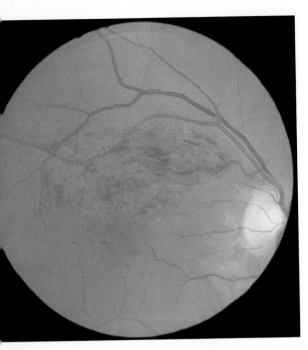

Plate 10.6 Right superotemporal fundus of patient with long-standing hypertension. There is marked retinal arteriosclerosis and a third-order superotemporal vein has become obstructed at an arteriovenous crossing just superior to the optic disc. The obstructed vein is tortuous and dilated and there is widespread intraretinal haemorrhage within its distribution, extending to involve the fovea.

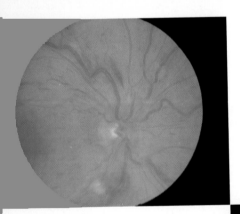

Plate 10.7 Right posterior fundus of patient with central retinal vein obstruction. The veins are grossly dilated and tortuous, and associated with perivascular haemorrhage and cotton wool spots.

Plate 10.8 Right posterior fundus of patient with advanced retinal vascular disease. There is widespread retinopathy, and a cilioretinal artery is occluded with macular ischaemia and a cherry red spot at the fovea.

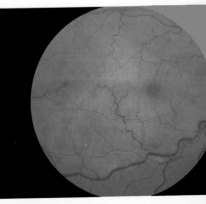

Plate 10.9a Left posterior pole of patient with background diabetic retinopathy. There are widespread microaneurysms, intraretinal haemorrhages and hard exudates (visual acuity 6/6).

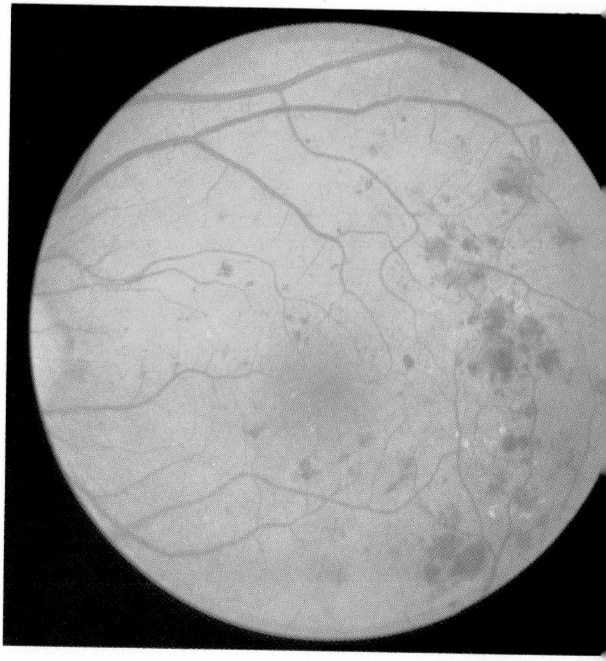

Plate 10.9b Fluorescein angiogram of fundus in (a), showing widespread microangiopathy and focal areas of non-perfused retina, temporal to left macula; defective superotemporal arteries stain with dye.

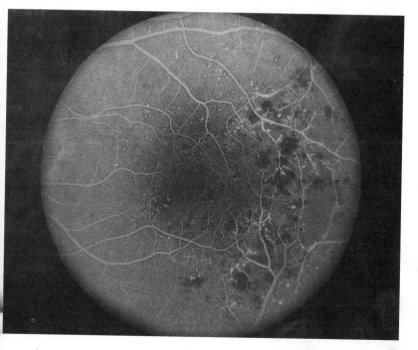

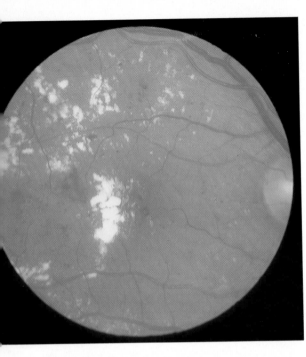

Plate 10.10 Right posterior fundus of patient with advanced background diabetic retinopathy and maculopathy. There are widespread microaneurysms and intraretinal haemorrhage. There is macular oedema with plaques of hard exudates encroaching on the right fovea (visual acuity 6/36).

Plate 10.11a (*bottom left*) Left superotemporal fundus of patient with proliferative diabetic retinopathy. Several foci of preretinal new vessels arise in the vicinity of major veins and ramify in the preretinal space. One focus shows evidence of sclerosis and involution.

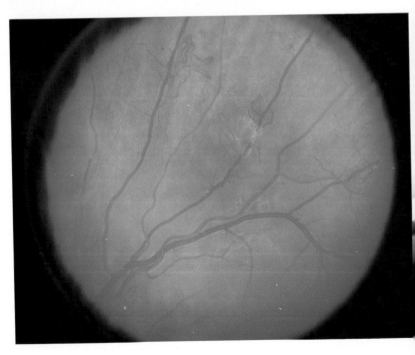

Plate 10.12 Left posterior fundus of patient with very probable toxocaral chorioretinitis. A discrete white proliferative chorioretinal lesion involves the macula, and the organizational process has resulted in a localized traction retinal detachment and temporal displacement of the major retinal vessels.

Plate 10.11b (*bottom right*) Venous phase angiogram of fundus in (a). There is widespread diabetic microangiopathy with extensive areas of non-perfused retina. The neovascular fronds are strikingly incompetent to dye and fluoresce brightly.

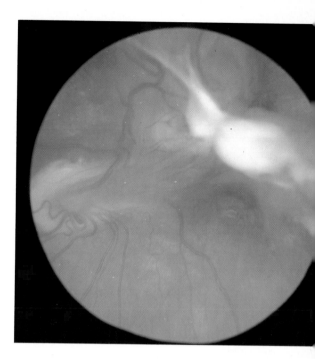

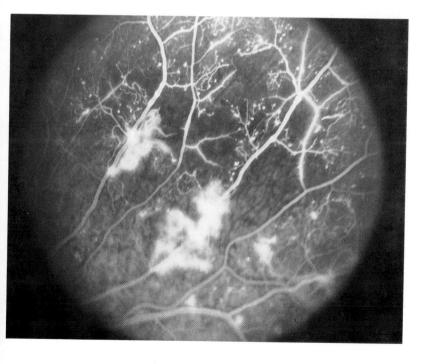

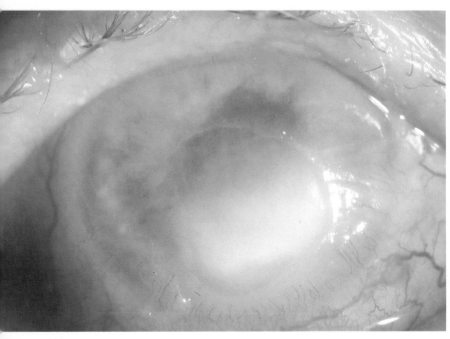

11.1a ▲

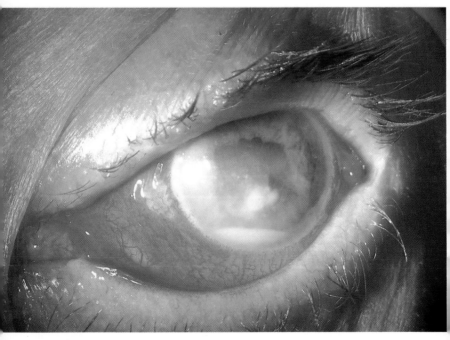

11.1b ▲

100 Basic Clinical Ophthalmology

Plate 11.1a Infected corneal ulcer, following abrasion by a tree branch while gardening.

Plate 11.1b Infected corneal ulcer with hypopyon. Note the fluid level, indicating pus which has gravitated to the lowest part of the anterior chamber. The infecting pneumococci came from an unsuspected low-grade inflammation in the tear sac which was due to blockage of the nasolacrimal duct; some mucopus regurgitated on syringing with lacrimal cannula.

Plate 11.2 Corneal abrasion stained with fluorescein eye drops, the excess 'washed off' with two or three drops of saline eyedrops.

Plate 12.1 Senile entropion.

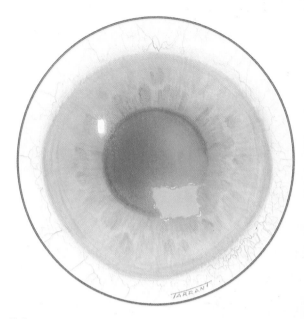

11.2 ▲

12.1 ▼

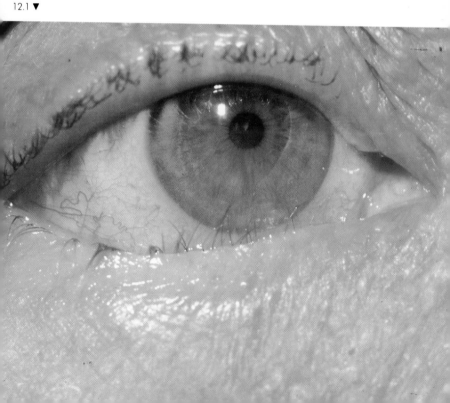

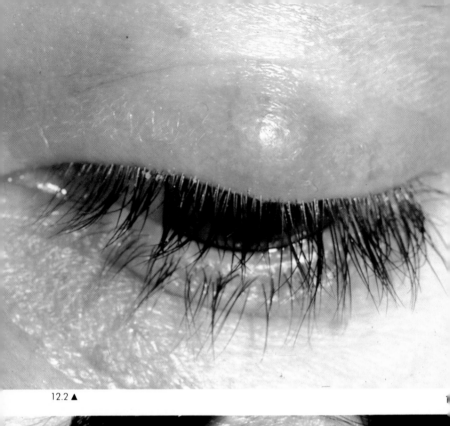

12.2 ▲

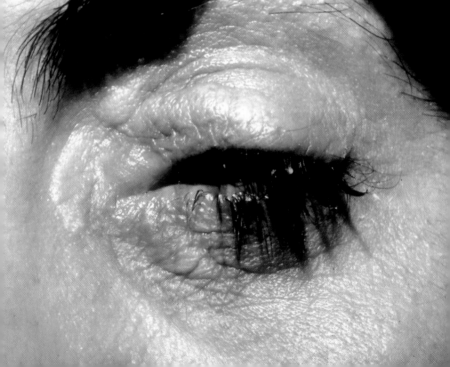

Plate 12.2 Internal hordeolum (acute chalazion)

Plate 12.3 Xanthelasmata.

Plate 13.1 Patient with left unilateral myopia (simulating proptosis) and divergent squint.

Plate 13.2 Upper lid retraction in thyrotoxicosis.

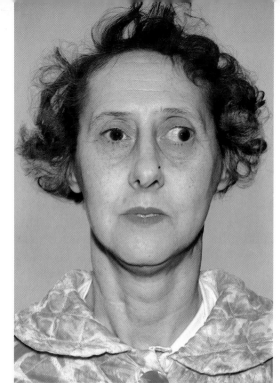

13.2 ▼   13.1 ▲

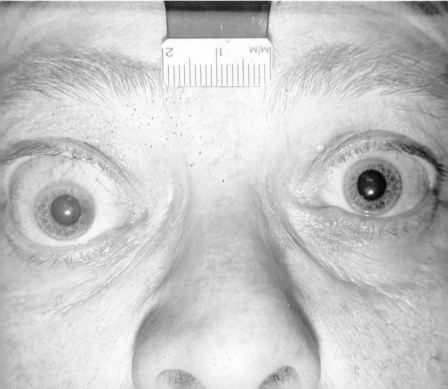

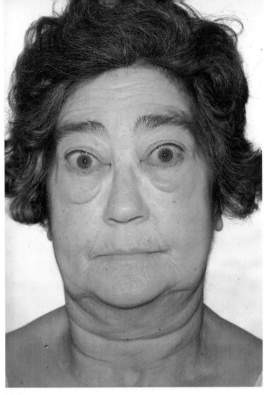

Plate 13.3 Patient with thyroid eye disease showing periorbital oedema, conjunctival injection, lid retraction and proptosis.

Plate 13.4 Patient with bilateral orbital cellulitis showing oedema, lid erythema and proptosis.

Plate 14.1 Filamentary keratitis after staining with Rose–Bengal.

Plate 14.2 Mucocele of the right lacrimal sac.

13.3 ▲

13.4 ◄

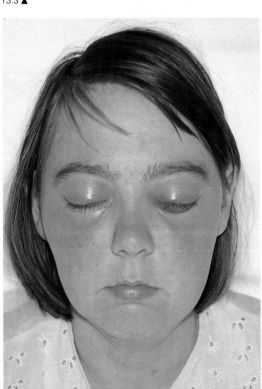

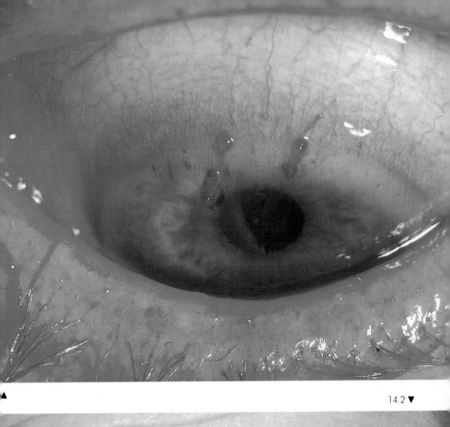

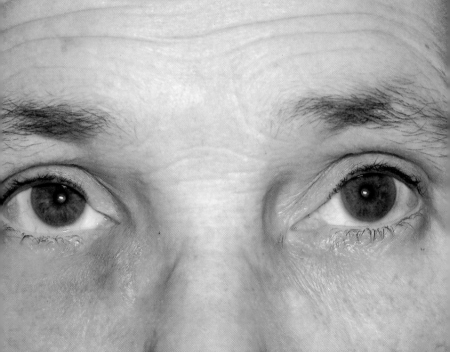

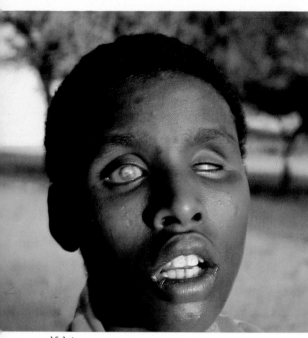

15.1 ▲

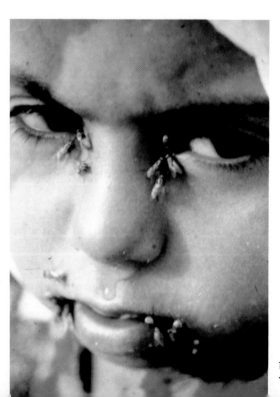

15.2
◄

Plate 15.1 Blind beggar boy aged 15 years. At the age of 3 years, vitamin A deficiency aggravated by measles produced keratomalacia. The right cornea is heavily scarred, hence only 'perception of light'. The left eyeball is shrunken after corneal perforation which failed to seal itself: no perception of light.

Plate 15.2 Moisture-seeking flies in a dry climate move quickly and indiscriminately from faeces to eyes of humans and animals (and food) and from eye to eye.

Plate 15.3 Pannus—i.e. vascularized fibrous tissue—invading the (upper) cornea, very typical of chronic trachoma.

Plate 15.4 Fibrosis (and neovascularization) well established under the hyperaemic conjuctiva covering the upper tarsal plate in an eye recurrently infected by the *Chlamydia trachomatis*.

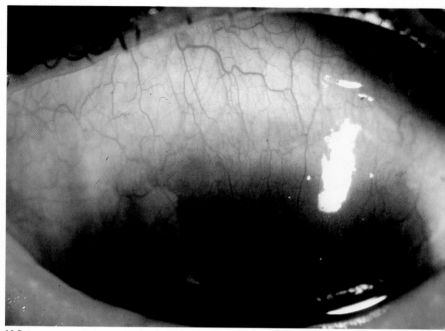

15.3

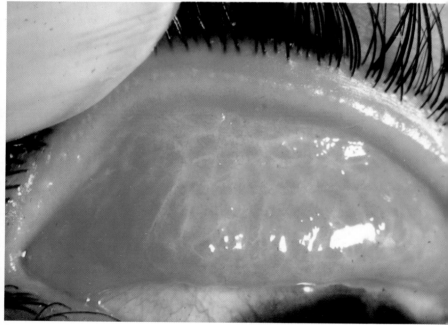

15.4 ▲

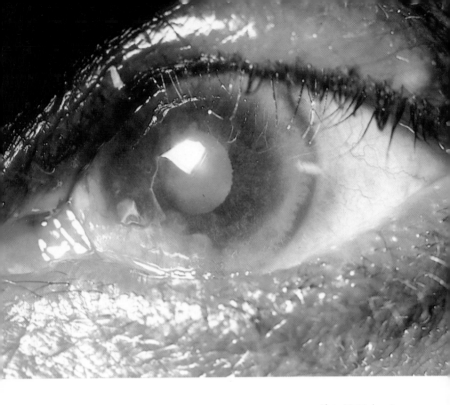

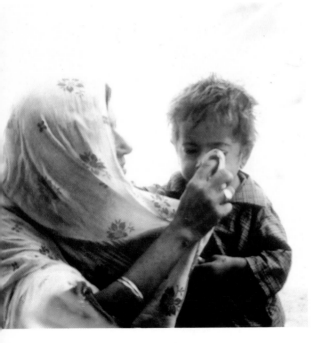

Plate 15.5 (*above*) Trichiasis. Contraction of fibrous tissue laid down in the eyelids and lid margins in response to recurrent infection by *Chlamydia trachomatis* for 10 years turns many eyelashes inwards to rub on the cornea. Corneal opacities are important causes of blindness in trachoma. Visual acuity in this (left) eye is 3/36. Cataract is also present.

Plate 15.6 (*left*) A Chadari used to wipe a child's eyes will form a reservoir to infect other children and reinfect this one.

Plate 15.7 (*right*) Close personal contact especially between children encourages the spread of *C. trachomatis* — and other infections.

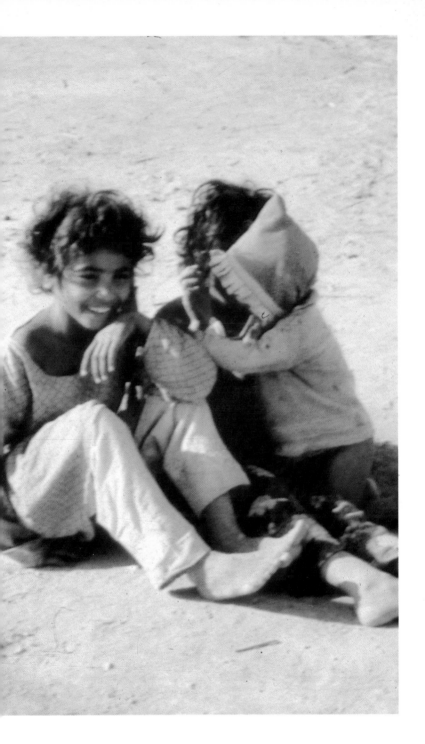

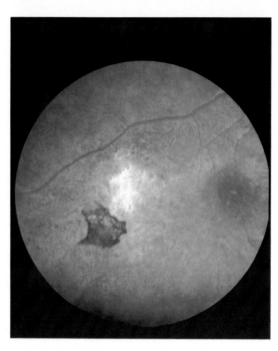

Plate 15.8 (*left*)
Onchocerciasis. Retinopathy, temporal to the macula. Atrophy of the pigment epithelium of the retina allows choroidal vessels to be visible.

Plate 15.9 (*below*)
Lepromatous leprosy. Bilateral lagophthalmos on attempted eyelid closure.

Plate 15.10 (*right*)
Lepromatous leprosy. Patches of iris atrophy.

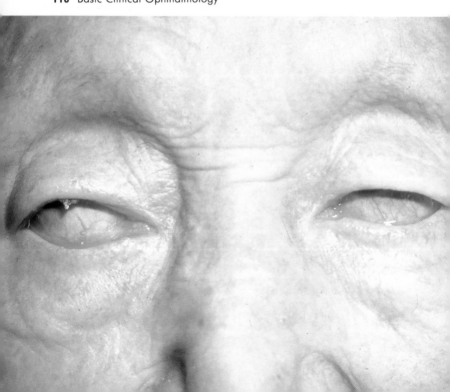

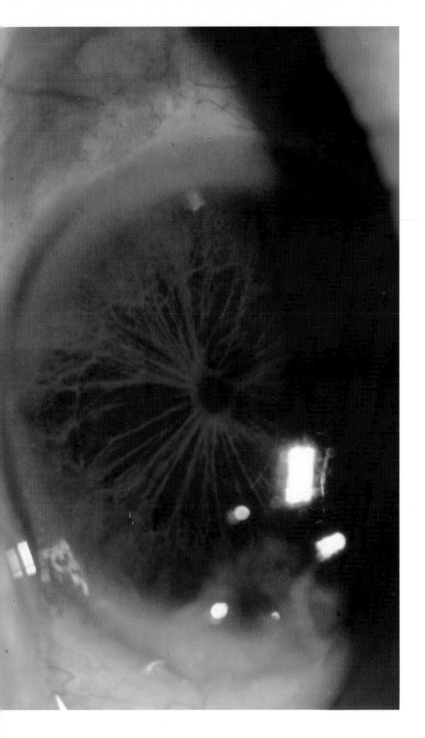

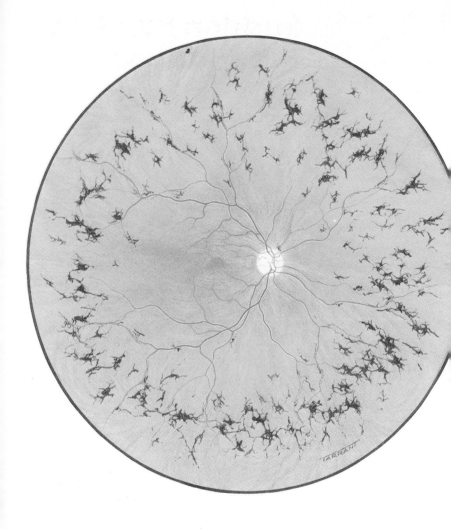

Plate 16.1 Typical fundus picture of established retinitis pigmentosa (*not* an inflammation of retina, in spite of the name). Note the pattern of pigmentation ('bone-corpuscle' because of a rather fanciful resemblance to this cell type), often obscuring retinal vessels, starting in equatorial region of the fundus and spreading forwards and backwards.

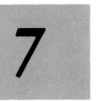

7 Sudden Painless Loss of Vision

S I Davidson and I Rennie

Introduction

The common causes of sudden painless visual loss in one eye can be attributed to acute loss of *retinal* function. The retina, an outgrowth of the central nervous system, has a high metabolic rate which is based almost exclusively upon aerobic respiration. Therefore disturbances in the blood supply to the retina (and nerve fibres forming the optic disc) have acute and profound effects upon visual function. The conditions capable of producing these circulatory changes include central retinal artery occlusion, transient occlusion of the central retinal artery (amaurosis fugax), central retinal vein occlusion, branch vein occlusion and giant cell (temporal) arteritis.

Applied anatomy

The central retinal artery is the major source of blood to the retina. This artery, a branch of the ophthalmic artery, enters the optic nerve 10–15 mm behind the globe and travels anteriorly within the nerve until it reaches the optic disc where it divides to form the major retinal branches. Retinal veins accompany these branches and join at the optic disc to form the central retinal vein. The central retinal vein enters the optic nerve at the optic disc and travels in close apposition to the central retinal artery throughout most of its course within the optic nerve. This intimate relationship of the central retinal artery and vein within the optic nerve is important when the pathogenesis of central retinal vein occlusion is considered (*see* below).

    The central retinal artery is an end-artery; that is, there is no anastomosis between its branches and any other system of vessels.

Whilst the branches of the central retinal artery supply the inner layers of the retina exclusively, the outer retinal layers (including the photoreceptors and retinal pigment epithelium) are nourished by the adjacent choroidal circulation.

The choroidal circulation is derived from between 10 and 20 small arteries which pierce the sclera at the posterior pole. These are called, rather confusingly, the short posterior ciliary arteries. Two or three of these vessels pierce the sclera close to the optic nerve and are responsible for the blood supply to the optic disc. Occlusion of one or more of these posterior ciliary vessels will deprive the nerve fibres which form the optic disc of their blood supply. This is of importance when considering the pathogenesis of the visual loss in giant cell (temporal) arteritis.

Central retinal artery occlusion

This is a rather uncommon cause of sudden visual loss.

Symptoms

The patient will complain of a sudden painless loss of vision in a previously healthy eye.

Signs

Visual acuity
Visual acuity will be significantly reduced in the affected eye to the level of counting fingers or worse. It is unusual for the vision to be completely extinguished (i.e. no perception of light).

The pupil in the affected eye will show a sluggish or absent response on direct light stimulation (afferent pupillary defect). It will, however, react normally to consensual stimulation.

Ophthalmoscopy will usually confirm the diagnosis. The ischaemic inner layers of the retina become oedematous and develop a pale milky appearance. This obscures the details of the choroidal circulation and retinal pigment epithelium which are normally just discernible. However, the reddish colour of the choroidal circulation is visible at the fovea, for the retina is normally thin in this region. The foveal appearance contrasts with the pallor of the surrounding retina to produce a cherry red spot (*see* Plate 7.1). Both arteries and veins, due to the absent or grossly reduced blood flow, appear attenuated and irregular in calibre. Occasionally, segmentation of the blood column is visible within the arteries (cattle trucking). It is useful to examine the healthy eye as a comparison if one is inexperienced in ophthalmoscopy. Furthermore, one must remember that the above changes are to some extent dependent on the duration of the occlusion. The signs may indeed be subtle if the fundus is examined immediately after the occlusion, before the development of the retinal oedema.

Pathogenesis

In common with other blood vessels, occlusion of the central retinal artery may be due to disease within the vessel itself or following embolization. In the elderly patient, retinal artery occlusion commonly follows thrombosis in an arteriosclerotic vessel. Indeed, as one would expect, there is an increased incidence of central retinal artery occlusion in patients with hypertension and systemic occlusive vascular disease. Inflammation within the artery wall may occasionally lead to its occlusion. (For this reason one should always be alert to the diagnosis of temporal arteritis as an infrequent but important cause of retinal artery occlusion; but *see* below.)

Emboli are a frequent cause of retinal artery occlusion, particularly in the younger patient. Common forms of emboli include platelets, calcium salts and cholesterol. The embolic material may be derived from an atheromatous internal carotid artery or from diseased heart valves. Auscultation over the carotid artery or precordium may reveal the source of the emboli.

Treatment

The treatment of central retinal artery occlusion is unsatisfactory. It is rare to obtain a return in retinal function after it has been deprived of its blood supply for more than a few minutes. If attempted, the methods of treatment are usually directed at improving retinal perfusion by lowering the intraocular pressure. Massage to the globe, anterior chamber paracentesis or intravenous administration of acetazolamide are occasionally used, with little effect upon the outcome. The most practical of these measures is *immediate* digital massage of the globe, which leads to reduction in intraocular pressure and, it is hoped, dislodgement of the embolus. It is more pertinent to look for a cause of the occlusion, rather than to attempt any form of treatment.

In this context one should always be alert to the diagnosis of temporal arteritis. Although this is an uncommon cause of sudden painless loss of vision, failure to diagnose and treat it risks total blindness because the untreated disease may become bilateral. This will be discussed at greater length in the section dealing with temporal arteritis.

Transient loss of vision in one eye (amaurosis fugax)

The occasional patient will present with a profound sudden loss of vision in one eye which lasts for a few seconds to a few minutes, full recovery in vision occurring within the next 20–30 minutes. The patient, in effect, is experiencing a transient ischaemic attack (TIA) affecting the retina. This symptom complex may be called amaurosis fugax. Microemboli, usually platelets, shed from a stenosed, atheromatous, internal carotid artery are the commonest cause of this phenomenon. Such an episode (or episodes) may be a harbinger of disaster: the patient often proceeds to develop a cerebral vascular occlusion within the territory of the diseased carotid artery.

Treatment

Amaurosis fugax, as the term implies, is self-limiting with a full recovery in retinal function. Again, particularly in the young patient, treatment, if contemplated, should be directed at the cause—e.g. the diseased carotid artery (aspirin to reduce platelet stickiness, anticoagulants or endarterectomy).

Central retinal vein occlusion

Symptoms

The patient again complains of a sudden painless loss of vision in the affected eye.

Signs

The vision is usually reduced to a level of 6/60 or less. Complete loss of vision (no perception of light) is rare in central retinal vein occlusion.

An afferent pupillary defect will usually accompany occlusion of the central retinal vein.

The fundal appearance is usually striking (*see* Plate 7.2). Multiple haemorrhages extending from the optic disc to the periphery of the retina are a prominent feature. The disc itself is often obscured by haemorrhages and oedema. The retinal haemorrhages, particularly those adjacent to the optic disc, are typically flame shaped; however, there is considerable variation in size and shape. Cotton wool spots, which are in fact small infarctions of the nerve fibre layer, are scattered throughout the retina. The retinal veins are tortuous, dilated and engorged with blood. Again, whilst this is the typical appearance, less extensive vein occlusions do occur.

Pathogenesis

Local and systemic factors may be involved in the development of a central retinal vein occlusion. The central retinal vein and artery, as described previously, are in close apposition within the optic nerve. Arteriosclerosis of the retinal artery will result in an increase in its diameter and subsequent compression of the retinal vein. This can be sufficient to initiate occlusion of the vein. It follows that widespread arterial disease and hypertension are both associated with central retinal vein occlusion. Increased viscosity of the blood associated with leukaemia, polycythaemia or dysgammaglobulinaemia may contribute to central retinal vein occlusion. The relationship between chronic simple glaucoma and central retinal vein occlusion is well established: approximately 20% of patients who develop central retinal vein occlusion have pre-existing glaucoma. Accordingly, a careful search must be made for open-angle and angle-closure glaucoma, especially in the fellow eye.

Treatment and prognosis

The prognosis for return of visual function in central retinal vein occlusion is variable. In a few cases some improvement in vision occurs, this being the exception rather than the rule. A number of therapeutic agents have been used in the treatment of central retinal vein occlusion. These include anticoagulants and fibrinolytic agents. Unfortunately, there is little evidence to support their use. It is again more important to exclude local and systemic causes for the occlusion. In particular it is important to remember that central retinal vein occlusion may occur in a previously undiagnosed case of glaucoma. Measurement of the intraocular pressures and assessment of the optic disc (in the fellow eye) and gonioscopy should be performed in all cases of central retinal vein occlusion.

Complications

The retinal ischaemia produced by the interruption of venous drainage will, in up to one-third of cases, stimulate the development of new blood vessels. This situation is analogous to the proliferative phase of diabetic retinopathy. Neovascularization may occur in sites other than the retina and optic disc, presumably because of diffusion of neovasculogenic substances. These include the anterior surface of the iris and trabecular meshwork. The new vessels present on the surface of the trabecular meshwork impede the drainage of aqueous from the eye, producing a secondary glaucoma (neovascular or rubeotic glaucoma). This type of glaucoma is typically painful and refractory to treatment. This situation may be avoided by performing prophylactic pan-retinal photocoagulation to convert ischaemic retina into 'dead' scar tissue. This will, in many cases, prevent the development of the new blood vessels.

Branch vein occlusion

It is more common for a branch vein to become occluded than for the central retinal vein to be involved. Ophthalmoscopy will reveal the signs of vein occlusion restricted to one quadrant of the retina. Visual acuity may be significantly reduced if the macula is involved but the prognosis is reasonable. It is uncommon for neovascularization to occur at a later date.

Giant cell (temporal) arteritis

This condition deserves special emphasis in the context of sudden painless visual loss. Giant cell (temporal) arteritis, as the name implies, is an inflammation of arteries which is not entirely restricted to the temporal arteries. It is more common than generally appreciated. Indeed, one post-mortem study demonstrated an incidence of approximately 1% in the population over 60 years of age.

Symptoms

The patient complains of a sudden visual loss in one eye. This is often associated with other symptoms, including headache, tenderness over the temporal arteries and general malaise. One particularly idiosyncratic symptom is pain on mastication due to claudication of the masseter muscle.

Signs

A profound visual loss is present. Complete loss of vision is not uncommon; i.e. there is 'no perception of light'. Initially one eye is usually involved *but there is grave danger of the fellow eye's being affected within a short period.*

Pupils
The direct light response is diminished or absent. The consensual light response is normal.

Ophthalmoscopy
This is dependent upon the distribution of the involved vessels. As stated previously, a central retinal artery occlusion may sometimes occur. However, it is more common for giant cell arteritis to involve the small posterior ciliary vessels which perfuse the optic disc (*see* 'Applied anatomy', above). Interruption of these vessels produces anoxia to the nerve fibres which form the optic disc. The resultant ischaemia produces localized oedema and swelling of the nerve fibres; clinically there is a pale waxy slightly elevated optic disc, typical of this 'ischaemic optic neuropathy'. Multiple splinter haemorrhages are present upon the oedematous disc. These signs to some extent mimic the changes that occur in papilloedema, but in the latter case the disc is hyperaemic. Indeed the term 'pale papilloedema' has been used to describe them. However, it is important to note that initially the fundus may have a normal appearance despite profound visual loss.

Pathogenesis

The diffuse arteritis possibly reflects an autoimmune response to elastic tissue in the blood vessels, resulting in small vessel occlusion.

Diagnosis

Confirmation of the diagnosis is obtained by finding a high ESR (e.g. 50 mm in 1 hour). In atypical cases temporal artery biopsy may assist the diagnosis when the ESR is not unduly elevated.

Treatment

Giant cell arteritis represents a true (ophthalmic) emergency. Whilst treatment will not aid recovery in the affected eye, it may prevent involvement of the fellow eye. *Tragically, it has been shown that, if untreated, a significant number of patients will develop a similar vascular occlusion in other eye—i.e. total bilateral blindness. This may occur within hours of the involvement of the first eye.* (We have seen a patient who lost the vision in the other eye whilst on his way to the pharmacy to collect his prescription!) *Systemic steroids in high doses will protect the vision in the remaining eye.* However, it is not sufficient to treat the patient initially with oral steroids alone. As soon as the diagnosis of giant cell arteritis is suspected, the patient should receive intravenous steroids even before being admitted to hospital. This should be followed by intramuscular steroids for the next 48 hours, *as well as* commencing oral therapy. The particular regimen used by the authors includes the administration of dexamethasone 4 mg intravenously followed by intramuscular dexamethasone 4 mg four times daily for 48 hours and at the same time prednisolone 60–80 mg by mouth daily. *It cannot be overemphasized that delay may result in irreversible blindness in both eyes.* The systemic steroid dosage may have to be maintained for months, but the dose should be gradually reduced after the first week towards a maintenance level at which the ESR remains normal.

8 Progressive Painless Loss of Vision

D L Easty

Painless, slowly progressive loss of vision is commonest in elderly patients. About 25% in Britain will be due to senile cataract and 25% to senile macular degeneration, and of course about 6% (25% × 25%) to both diseases. Two other important causes—glaucoma (16%) and diabetic retinopathy (7%) are discussed in Chapters 5 and 10, respectively. For some neurological causes, *see* Chapter 9.

An exacting history is helpful in assessing the patient who has noticed that his vision is deteriorating painlessly, in whom there is no improvement when he visits his optician. In many cases of slowly progressive visual loss, the patient may not be aware of the deficit, especially if only one eye is affected, or is predominantly affected. His attention may be drawn to it by some chance event, or indeed as a result of a routine eye test. The loss of vision may seemingly be sudden. Diseases which affect the optic media may be noticed at an early stage particularly in bright light. On the other hand, a partial retinal detachment when it first occurs may be dismissed as unimportant because it affects peripheral vision rather than the central field. In disease of the central nervous system—for example, in expanding lesions in the pituitary fossa or where the optic nerve is compressed by an expanding intracranial neoplasm—the loss of vision may be subtle and remain unnoticed.

Initial complaints are important because they provide information about the cause of the visual loss. For example, in early cataract or in corneal disease where the stroma is involved, there can be scattering of light and the patient may complain that the symptoms are particularly noticeable when driving at night, when the headlamps of oncoming traffic cause glare and sometimes multiple images.

Examination

This should follow the routine which has already been described (Chapter 2). Lens opacities can be seen with an ophthalmoscope (*see* Plate 8.1). Their presence is not necessarily serious and they may not always be the cause of visual loss, particularly if they are not situated on the visual axis. Opacities which occur in the cortex are often wedge-shaped (*cuneiform*) and are not always very significant. It is when opacities occur in the centre of the posterior surface of the lens—when they are called *posterior subcapsular lens opacities*—that considerable visual loss can occur in spite of the fact that the clinical appearances would belie this.

Often in the elderly, senile miosis (which is physiological) prevents ophthalmoscopy, particularly if there are early lens opacities. Mydriasis can be obtained with drops such as tropicamide 0.5% or 1.0% (Mydriacyl) or cyclopentolate 1% (Mydrilate). This gives the observer the satisfaction of reaching an accurate diagnosis. Other diseases involving the posterior segment, such as macular disease or chronic simple glaucoma, can then be excluded. It should be remembered that in the elderly it is not unusual for more than one disease process to be active within the eye.

It can be a worry when no positive findings are made in the eye to account for loss of vision. Examination then should include an evaluation of the pupillary reactions to light and for near, looking for evidence of an afferent pupillary deficit. This might provide evidence of a lesion in the central nervous system. Visual fields can be effectively assessed using confrontation techniques (Chapter 2). When the technique is used with both eyes open, a lack of awareness of movement on one side when moving both hands simultaneously ('inattention hemianopia') provides evidence of an *orientation* defect, which can be the cause of apparent loss of vision, in the presence of seemingly normal fields using standard techniques.

The cornea

Anatomy

The cornea is a unique tissue by virtue of its physical characteristics. It is transparent and avascular and has considerable tensile strength, and acts as a lens. It is the most powerful refractive element within the visual system because of the large difference between the refractive index of air and cornea (the difference between aqueous humour and lens is much less). The adult cornea is oval with a horizontal diameter of 12 mm and a vertical diameter of 11 mm. The centre of the cornea is approximately 0.5 mm in thickness.

It can be divided into five separate layers: (1) the anterior corneal epithelial and basement membrane; (2) Bowman's membrane; (3) the stroma; (4) Descemet's membrane; and (5) the endothelium. The epithelium is composed of five or six layers of squamous cells. Bowman's membrane is acellular and made of collagen fibres, and is about 10–16 μm thick. The stroma comprises about 90% of the total thickness and is composed of keratocytes, which are thought to be a special form of fibrocyte, found between bundles of collagen fibres. The extracellular space contains proteoglycans, salts and water. The collagen fibres are equal in diameter and also are equidistant from each other. This arrangement forms an ordered array or matrix which is said to account in part for the transparency of the cornea. Descemet's membrane has a smooth, glass-like appearance and is approximately 8–10 μm in thickness. The endothelium is a single layer of cells that lines the posterior surface of the cornea, and is in contact with aqueous humour. The cells of this layer have high metabolic activity, as shown by their rich endoplasmic reticulum. Its role is to pump fluid from the cornea into the anterior chamber, as it is well known that blocking the function of this layer results in corneal swelling and loss of transparency.

Corneal disease

A disturbance in the central cornea within its structure or on its surface will reduce the visual acuity. The tear film maintains a perfectly smooth refractive surface. Chronic abnormality of this film, as in patients with poor secretion of tears, leads to reduction of vision. The common disturbances of the corneal epithelium and stroma are due to infection (Chapter 6) or injury (Chapter 11, especially Plates 11.1 a and b) or, less commonly, are the result of hereditary disease (Chapter 16).

All the important layers of the cornea may be affected by progressive disease. Calcium may be deposited in Bowman's layer in the exposed area of cornea which lies between the lids—when it is called *band-shaped keratopathy* (*see* Plate 8.2). It may be secondary to uveitis, glaucoma or chronic disease leading to collapse of the globe (phthisis bulbi). It can be seen with hypercalcaemia, hypophosphatasia or uraemia. The deposit can be removed with chelating agents plus the help of a spatula.

Stromal dystrophies are bilaterally symmetrical, avascular, inherited affections of the cornea which may be accompanied by systemic disease (Table 8.1). Most dystrophies have presented by the second decade. They are relatively rare, the commonest being lattice dystrophy which is Mendelian dominant and presents towards the end of the first decade. The changes generally occur in the anterior part of the stroma in the central region (*see* Plate 8.3).

Disease category	Diagnosis	Observations
Epithelial disease: Band keratopathy	Calcified opaque band in exposed area of cornea	Associated with chronic inflammatory disease of the eye, and endocrine or renal disease affecting calcium metabolism. Deposit can be removed
Keratoconjunctivitis sicca	Poor tear secretion produces epithelial disease of cornea and conjunctiva. Visual blurring because of abnormal tear film	May be associated with rheumatoid arthritis (Sjögren's syndrome). Treat with artificial tears
Stromal inflammatory disease	Progressive visual loss due to corneal clouding—many causes, e.g. herpes simplex and zoster keratitis	Usually associated with pain or photophobia, or a history of acute inflammatory disease
Corneal dystrophies: Granular	Fine granular stromal opacities. Visual acuity affected late in life	Dominant
Lattice	A fine lattice plus diffuse central opacity	Dominant
Macular	Rare—isolated stromal opacities with little influence on vision	Recessive
Ectatic conditions (keratoconus)	Conical cornea, which distorts the lower lid when patient looks down. Associated with central corneal thinning	Initially can be treated with contact lens, with good visual return. May eventually require penetrating keratoplasty
Corneal oedema: Bullous keratopathy	Common. Follows intra-ocular surgery. Diffuse corneal opacification	Occasional sharp pain. Penetrating keratoplasty may be required
Endothelial dystrophy	Variable visual blurring and diffuse stromal and epithelial oedema. Rare	Penetrating keratoplasty required
Neurotrophic keratitis	Trigeminal nerve palsy; associated with facial anaesthesia. Gradual visual blurring due to inflammatory disease and secondary infection	Full investigation and treatment in eye department
Exposure keratitis	Induced by poor lid closure—e.g. due to facial nerve palsy. Epithelial breakdown and possible secondary infection producing corneal scarring	Surgical repair when due to lid disease; partial lid closure (tarsorrhaphy) when facial palsy
Keratomalacia	Visual loss due to epithelial and stromal disease	Improved on treatment of vitamin-A-deficient patient

Table 8.1 Painless progressive loss of vision due to corneal disease

Endothelial dystrophies occur in elderly patients, but are uncommon. Fuchs' dystrophy is the least rare. The endothelial pump ceases to function, and the stroma becomes waterlogged; blisters or bullae occur in the epithelium which cause pain when they rupture—'*bullous keratopathy*', which may also follow intraocular operations where the endothelium has been damaged. *The endothelial layer has minimal or no ability to regenerate.*

Corneal grafting

Where the corrected vision drops to a level of less than 6/36 as a result of a corneal opacity and the patient is sufficiently incapacitated, then a corneal graft (keratoplasty) can be done. A disc of cornea, usually 7–8 mm in diameter and including the diseased area, is trephined out of the patient's eye and replaced by a disc from a donor eye removed by the same trephine. The disc may be full thickness or, if the opacity is superficial, only half or three-quarters thickness. The new tissue usually remains transparent and provides useful return of sight (*see* Plate 8.4). Donor corneal tissue is often difficult to obtain and the general practitioner can often help in advising patients about the value of corneal grafting. The methods of eye donation can be found out by contacting the local eye surgeons or the administrators of the eye hospital.

The lens

The lens is a unique tissue in the body because it is transparent and avascular, similar to the cornea, but achieving its transparency by a seemingly different mechanism. It contains a high concentration of protein (35%) when compared with other biological tissues found in nature. It contributes less to the refracting system of the eye than does the cornea. It is isolated from the immune system of the body from early embryonic life; in later life, should lens matter be released into the cavity of the eye and the circulation, its protein may act as antigenic 'not-self' or 'foreign' material.

Embryologically, surface ectoderm covering the primitive optic cup invaginates during the first three weeks of gestation (*see* Chapter 1 and Plate 1.3). Cells that are destined to become the anterior lens epithelium continue to secrete basement membrane, which eventually surrounds the external surface of the lens epithelium, forming the lens capsule which is impermeable to the immune system of the body. The cells in the posterior part of the embryonic lens vesicle elongate in an anterior–posterior manner to form the primary lens fibres which eventually compose the embryonal nucleus.

The lens is biconvex and is located in the anterior segment between the iris anteriorly and the anterior vitreous face posteriorly. The central part of the posterior surface is known as the posterior pole, and the edge of the lens is the equator. The diameter in adults is 9.0 mm while the anterior–posterior thickness is 3.5–4.0 mm. The lens continues to enlarge throughout life (Fig 8.1). Beneath the capsule is the lens epithelium, which anteriorly is a single

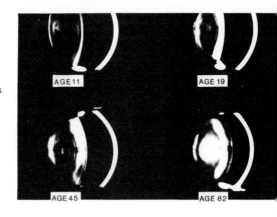

Fig 8.1 The development of the lens in a normal subject. The lens continues to expand throughout life and produces some shallowing of the anterior chamber in the elderly. (Courtesy of Nicholas Brown.)

cuboidal layer of cells interdigitating with and attached to each other by desmosomal connections. Golgi complexes are located in the posterior portion of the cell, which are probably responsible for the capsule formation in embryonic life. The epithelium in the pre-equatorial zone undergoes mitotic division, inwards migration and considerable elongation to form lens fibres. The process of laying down of fibres occurs continuously so that the originally superficial epithelial cells at the equator become more deeply situated. These fibres may then constitute the cortex of the lens. Each of the fibres of the cortex has a cell nucleus and nucleolus as well as cytoplasmic polyribosome chains that manufacture the proteins of the lens, e.g. α-, β-, and γ-crystallins. In addition to mitochondria there are microtubules, but few Golgi complexes or endoplasmic reticulum. The absence of these latter organelles suggests that lens protein is not secreted into the extracellular environment but is retained within the cytoplasm.

Proceeding from the cortex towards the centre of the lens, the morphology changes. Nuclei become fragmented and finally disappear, and the intracellular organelles decrease. The core of the lens demonstrates fragmented cell membranes with a dense homogenous cytoplasm. There is no intercellular space between adjacent fibres. The constant process of catabolism and anabolism that protein undergoes throughout the body would not seem to be possible in the core, where there is little scientific evidence of overt protein synthesis because of the absence of appropriate cell machinery. Protein in this part is synthesized during embryogenesis and is able to remain stable for 60 or more years and for the most part retains transparency. It is often this part of the lens which loses its transparency in old age, possibly because of the relative lack of protein renewal.

Cataract

'Cataract' refers to any opacity occurring within the normally transparent lens. It is an emotive term and so should be used with caution in front of

Age of onset	Congenital
	Infantile
	Juvenile
	Adult
	Senile
Anatomical site	Cortical
	Nuclear
	Capsular (anterior or posterior)
	Subcapsular (anterior or posterior)
Development	Stationary
	Progressive
Degree of opacity	Immature
	Mature

Table 8.2 Classifications of cataract

patients. Cataracts can occur in the newborn (congenital), infants, juveniles, and adults but very much more commonly in the elderly (Table 8.2). The nucleus, cortex, capsular or subcapsular regions can be involved. They are often described as immature when there are transparent lens fibres present, and mature when the entire lens becomes opaque. However, the latter is not a useful classification today, although it used to be important; it does not help particularly in making decisions about cataract removal which now depends on visual function and incapacity. In the early days of cataract surgery, it was easier to remove mature or hypermature lenses, so the degree of visual handicap prior to the operation must have been much more than it is in cataract patients today. By no means all cataracts are progressive. Cataract is seen in association with a number of systemic disorders (Table 8.3).

Congenital cataracts
These may arise from many causes and may become manifest and progress after birth (*see* Plate 8.5). They may be isolated or be associated with systemic disorders. The opacities may be subtle and hardly apparent, with no significant effect on vision, or they may be so advanced that the pupil is white. There may be a positive family history. The infant may present with a history of poor visual development. A history of maternal infection by rubella or cytomegalovirus during the first trimester has been a significant cause in the past. Inborn metabolic disturbances such as galactosaemia, diabetes mellitus, hypoparathyroidism and homocysteinuria can be associated with

Disease	Lenticular changes	Investigations
No associated disease:		
Congenital	Many forms: lamellar, coralliform, punctate	Nil
Adult		
Senile	Cortical, posterior, subcapsular or nuclear Occur above 70 years: nuclear, cortical and posterior subcapsular	Exclude local ocular disease and systemic disease such as diabetes mellitus
Metabolic disease:		
Diabetes mellitus	Increased incidence and more rapid maturation of senile cataract in diabetics. True diabetic cataract rare; subcapsular snowstorm opacities—which partially clear with treatment	Urine tests and fasting blood sugar estimation
Galactosaemia	Initial anterior and posterior subcapsular opacity in infancy	Test for raised blood and urine galactose levels
Hypocalcaemia	Dot subcapsular opacities eventually become lamellar cataracts	Associated with infantile tetany, hypoparathyroidism and cretinism. Serum calcium depressed
Hereditary cataract in association with:		
Renal disease (Lowe's syndrome)	Congenital cataract; hyperplastic anterior capsule; posterior capsule adherent to vitreous	Mental retardation, amino-aciduria, tubular acidosis, dwarfism, rickets
Skeletal disease (Marfan's syndrome)	Cataract as well as lens subluxation	Associated with typical skeletal abnormalities; homocysteinuria should be excluded
Chromosomal disorders (Down's syndrome)	Cataract develops towards the end of first decade of life. Congenital lens opacities often present	Chromosome studies
Non-hereditary cataract (rubella syndrome)	Cataract may be advanced and associated with other ocular disease (e.g. glaucoma)	Serum antibody titre against rubella; many other systemic associations (e.g. deafness, cardiac abnormalities)
Cataract associated with isolated ocular defects	Variable	Ocular conditions in association: microphthalmia, aniridia, retinitis pigmentosa, intraocular inflammation, absolute glaucoma, retinal detachment
Traumatic cataract	Associated with ruptured capsule due to penetrating injury. Contusion injury may induce posterior subcapsular opacity	Exclude intraocular foreign body by x-ray
Toxic cataract	Systemic or topical cortico-steroid for long periods may cause posterior subcapsular cataract. Also ergot, naphthalene	

Disease	Lenticular changes	Investigation
Electromagnetic radiation:		
Infrared	Posterior cortical cataract in glass workers	
Ionizing radiation	Granular opacity in the posterior capsule and subcapsular region. May advance to maturity	
Ultraviolet	Little evidence of industrial association. Possible association with senile cataract	

Table 8.3   Cataract associated with other disease

cataract. In rheumatoid arthritis in children (oligoarticular) the associated anterior uveitis can induce secondary cataract formation (*see* Plate 8.6).

Acquired cataract
This may be hereditary in origin and may be progressive. The senile type (Fig 8.2) is increasingly common with the longer life spans which occur today. Senile cataract accounts for much of the surgery which is performed by ophthalmologists, and is an interesting and rewarding field. Diabetes mellitus represents a strong risk factor. There is some evidence of an association with high blood pressure and relatively high blood sugar (diabetes excluded) [1, 2]. A few toxic substances can cause cataract. For example, psoralens are drugs used in the treatment of (severe) psoriasis, being given by mouth. After absorption the drug is deposited in the skin and, unfortunately, in the lens of the eye. Exposure to ultraviolet light, which is absorbed by the psoralens, improves the skin but will produce cataract unless appropriate protective goggles are worn continuously for 24 hours after ingestion of the psoralens.

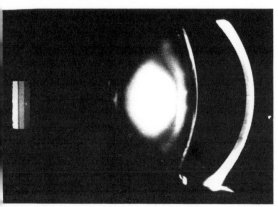

Fig 8.2 A slit-lamp photograph showing central nuclear lens opacities which substantially reduce vision. The cornea is the bright isolated dome to the right.

Symptoms

Symptoms of senile cataract are of a gradual decrease of vision which is not associated with pain or inflammation, except where cataract occurs secondarily to chronic uveitis. Multiple images may occur, and vision may sometimes be improved where the environmental illumination is reduced, due to a partial dilatation of the pupil. In nuclear cataracts there is a slowly progressive change in refraction towards myopia. Lens opacities may be caused by toxic compounds such as certain of the phenothiazines (*see* Plate 8.7) which are comparatively mild, but more severe opacities follow the use of systemic or topical corticosteroid. The lens opacities are situated in the posterior subcapsular region of the lens. Peripheral cortical opacities may look rather spoke-like when they are seen early, but gradually they expand to form wedges which may coalesce to produce diffuse opacities (*see* Plate 8.1). The presence of cortical opacities does not necessarily cause impaired vision, and they can remain almost static for years.

Treatment

Conservative treatment should be the policy of choice as long as possible. When the patient has symptoms which cause him significant incapacity or handicap, which usually means that he can no longer perform his work, or that he cannot read small print, then a decision to remove the cataract must be made. A fall, or trip over an irregularity in the pavement may be a sign that the patient needs cataract extraction to prevent more serious mishaps such as hip fracture. It is at a corrected visual acuity of 6/36 for distance that the ability to read normal print deteriorates. A decision to operate depends upon requirements and occupation; most surgeons remove the more advanced cataract when the corrected vision in the better eye is 6/18 or 6/24, or worse. Up to this stage, the patient is refracted to ensure that his spectacle correction is accurate; it is surprising how much the vision can be helped with a change of glasses in many patients.

UNILATERAL CATARACT

After removal of a unilateral cataract, optical correction with a very strong spectacle lens (+10 dioptre sphere usually) causes a 25% enlargement of the image, so that fusion of the images from the two eyes cannot take place, and diplopia occurs. It is because of this difficulty that the advances made in contact lenses, as well as the development of intraocular implants, have made it more acceptable to remove a unilateral cataract and so retrieve binocular vision.

Depending on the age, general health and occupation requirements of the patient, most surgeons will remove the worse of the two cataracts first; then, some weeks or months later, the cataract in the second eye. Some favour operation on both eyes at the same session. Others avoid operation on the second eye, at least in the elderly and/or infirm, unless hypermaturity is a danger. Intraocular lens implants are being increasingly used (*see* below).

Operations for cataract

The student should try to attend the operation theatre to see one of the most elegant and satisfying operations in the whole of surgery. Local or general anaesthesia is used. An incision into the eyeball at the limbus (corneoscleral junction) is made, from about 10 to 2 o'clock, to achieve access to the cataractous lens. A preliminary limbus-based flap of conjunctiva plus Tenon's capsule is usually made so that the limbal wound will heal more quickly and securely, and so that the five to ten fine sutures in the incision at the corneoscleral junction are buried at the end of the operation when the flap is sutured back into place. Another common feature is a peripheral or sector iridectomy. Thereafter, either the intracapsular or extracapsular method is employed: both are unfortunate names.

In the *intracapsular* extraction the whole lens is removed along with, and within, its capsule. The suspensory ligament of the lens may be digested enzymatically by α-chymotrypsin (Zonulysin) and the lens is removed using a cryoprobe at −60 to −30°C. The very cold tip of the probe freezes to the surface of the lens, which can then be gently rocked out of the eye. The original incision is closed with fine sutures, and the conjunctival flap is sewn back into place.

In the *extracapsular* cataract extraction, the surface of the anterior capsule of the lens is incised with a cystotome, so that a central disc of capsule can be removed. The nucleus of the lens is squeezed very gently upwards, starting with pressure at 6 o'clock on the corneoscleral margin, along with some simultaneous manoeuvres made directly through the incision, usually with the cystotome. Residual 'lens matter' is thoroughly irrigated out of the eye with a special physiological-saline-based solution. The posterior lens capsule is left behind and acts as a barrier between the anterior segment and posterior segment, thus reducing the risk of vitreous loss, which can be a hazard in the intracapsular technique.

Complications

In cataract surgery complications do occur but are rather uncommon because of improved surgical technique, especially the use of the operation microscope. One of the most important complications is vitreous loss, which increases the risk of subsequent retinal detachment.

Prolapse of iris tissue through the incision can occur, which can be dangerous, and is an indication for immediate action (iridectomy) by the eye surgeon. Bleeding occasionally occurs from the corneoscleral incision, to produce a hyphaema (blood in the anterior chamber). Any suggestion of infection manifesting as persistent redness, pain, lid swelling and the appearance of pus in the anterior chamber, with a fluid level, is an indication for immediate referral. The interior of the eye at the early stages of infection is privileged from the immune system, and so this makes it all the more important that appropriate investigations and therapy be urgently applied.

Patients who have had cataracts removed may be treated with aphakic spectacles. The correction of aphakia requires high plus (convex) spectacle lenses. These lenses may have aberrations which cause difficulty for the patient, in addition to which there is approximately 25% enlargement of image size. A ring scotoma occurs as a result of the prismatic effect of the lens periphery. The effective field is restricted, and patients may suffer from initial insecurity and poor balance with their new spectacles. When lenses are fitted close to the eye, have a full aperture and are aspherical they can provide a better field of vision. The distortion of the central image can be reduced with aspheric lenses. Contact lenses can be fitted, which may be hard or soft, but the elderly find them difficult to manage. Soft lenses can be retained for several days without removal (intermediate wear contact lenses). These will reduce the magnification and ring scotoma from spectacle lenses which can be the cause of so many problems for these patients. Intraocular lens implants (*see* below), especially in unilateral cataract and aphakia, allow the patient to avoid most of these problems, but with some risk of others.

Unilateral aphakia
This creates a disparity in the images seen by spectacle correction, which cannot be tolerated. The usual cause is a traumatic cataract due to penetrating injury but it may also occur in the elderly when one eye is affected and operated on before the other. A contact lens may solve the difficulty. An additional problem arises in unilateral cataract in the newborn or in children under, say, 3–4 years (in the latter, usually due to injury). 'Deprivation amblyopia'—compare 'suppression amblyopia' in strabismus—will occur quickly and permanently unless operation is done within a few days or week or two of birth or injury, *and* unless a contact lens can be consistently worn or an intraocular lens inserted.

Intraocular lens implants
These are used by a majority of surgeons especially for patients with

unilateral cataract, but also for the elderly with bilateral cataract. They are clear plastic lenses manufactured from acrylic material (polymethylmethacrylate). The common feature of the many varieties is, of course, the siting of the actual lenses in the pupil area. Some surgeons favour those lenses which are positioned just anterior to the plane of the pupil, supported by 'legs' resting in the angle of the anterior chamber. Others prefer those lenses just behind the plane of the pupil, supported by 'legs' usually resting in the recess immediately behind the base of the iris, between it and the ciliary body proper. Popular as these lenses are with patients and surgeons, a penalty of their use is a small increase in the rate of postoperative complications; for example, the merest contact between lens and corneal endothelium at the time of operation may well result in damage to the endothelium which may cause permanent corneal oedema and loss of vision years later.

The retina

Macular degeneration

The macular area of the retina is situated opposite the pupil, has a high density of cones and has been designed by Nature (!) to see fine detail; the peripheral retina has less densely packed rods so that it can register only grosser images (see Chapter 1).

Selective diseases of the cones at the macula may occur at any age and are often hereditary; all are uncommon except senile macular degeneration (Table 8.4). Selective disease of peripheral retina may also occur; for example, retinitis pigmentosa (see Chapter 16) which spares the macular area, at least until late in the disease. Interestingly, since developmentally the retina is really part of the brain, some retinal dystrophies are associated with CNS—or other—diseases; for example, amaurotic familial idiocy (Tay–Sachs disease)—i.e. GM_2 gangliosidosis type I [3] and Bassen–Kornzweig syndrome which is retinitis pigmentosa associated with abetalipoproteinaemia.

Senile macular degeneration

This eventually produces bilateral central scotomas, leaving the patient unable to read or recognize faces; he can be encouraged by being told that he will always retain his peripheral fields and so be able to cross roads, etc. Ophthalmoscopically, a gradually increasing and extending pigment disturbance, first at the fovea centralis (the centre of the macular area), can be seen if the pupil is dilated by a mydriatic (see Plate 8.8). It is

Associated with neurological disease

Amaurotic family idiocy:

Tay–Sachs disease	Cherry red spot
Late infantile	Bull's eye retinopathy
Juvenile	Bull's eye maculopathy
Niemann–Pick disease	Cherry red spot

Unassociated with neurological disease

Involving:

Photoreceptors and pigment epithelium:

Cone (-rod) dystrophy	Bull's eye maculopathy
Stargardt's disease	Atrophic macula surrounded by yellow flecks
Pericentric retinitis pigmentosa	Bone corpuscle pigmentation around perimacular vessels
Progressive atrophic macular dystrophy	Atrophic macular lesion in second–third decade

Retinal pigment epithelium:

Vitelliform dystrophy	Egg-yellow elevated circular structure
Fundus flavimaculatus	Yellowish irregular spots over posterior poles
Dominant drüsen	Multiple drüsen
Reticular dystrophy	Macular pigment granules; peripheral reticular deposits

Bruch's membrane:

Pseudoinflammatory dystrophy	Oedema, haemorrhages and exudates
Angioid streaks	Greyish lines radiating from disc; macular degeneration (sometimes disciform)
Senile macular dystrophy	Pleomorphic
Myopic degeneration	Pleomorphic. Often haemorrhagic

Choroid: central choroidal atrophy	Sharply defined area of pigment epithelial atrophy with disappearance of choriocapillaris

sometimes preceded by a multiplicity of yellow spots called drüsen, due to colloid deposits under the pigment epithelium (*see* Plate 8.9). Myopia is a predisposing factor. The best guess at aetiology is a hereditary degenerative process in the cones.

At any stage, a subretinal haemorrhage may occur, wrecking the cones, because one reaction to the degenerative process is the growth of fragile new vessels from the underlying choroid through Bruch's membrane and the pigment epithelium. 'Senile *disciform* macular degeneration' has now occurred, and a plaque of organized fibrous tissue results. That particular complication may be preventable by light coagulation (usually by argon laser) of these new vessels, rendered visible by fluorescein fundus photography, provided they are more than 200 μm from the fovea. Iatrogenic loss of vision usually occurs if vessels within that radius are treated—or indeed if too much heat is applied to vessels beyond that limit. However, the underlying degenerative process probably continues.

Chloroquine retinopathy

This constitutes an iatrogenic macular degeneration. It occurs in patients with rheumatoid arthritis because the dosage of chloroquine is much greater than is used prophylactically or therapeutically in malaria. The drug accumulates at the macular area to cause a little ring scotoma at first around the fixation point, followed by gradual reduction in central vision. The dose should be at or below a daily average of 200 mg chloroquine for rheumatoid arthritis (half of that for disseminated lupus erythematosus) with a maximum of 75 g per annum up to a grand total dose of 300 g; regular monitoring throughout, especially if these doses are exceeded, is indicated [4, 5].

Central serous retinopathy

In this rather uncommon condition which affects the macula, there is an accumulation of serous fluid between the pigment epithelium and the rods and cones. The cause is quite unknown. The macula becomes elevated, and visual acuity is reduced usually only to 6/18 or so. Patients between 25 and 40 years are affected, usually males. Recovery from the disorder usually occurs spontaneously in between 2 and 4 months. It is generally unilateral. Fluorescein angiography may demonstrate one or two points of leakage through the retinal pigment epithelium of choroidal extracellular fluid. These can be sealed by laser treatment. It is difficult to see retinal oedema with the direct ophthalmoscope; the foveal reflex disappears, and a tell-tale circle of light reflex circumscribing the macula may be enough for the diagnosis to be made.

Cystoid macular oedema

This is a term used to denote oedema resulting from leakage of fluid (from the retinal capillaries) which infiltrates the retinal layers around the macular region. It is seen clearly with fluorescein angiography, which shows a petalloid appearance (Fig 8.3). There are a large number of causes, the most important being a previous cataract extraction, glaucoma filtering surgery, diabetic retinopathy, branch retinal vein occlusion and uveitis. Fortunately, the condition often clears up spontaneously; but it

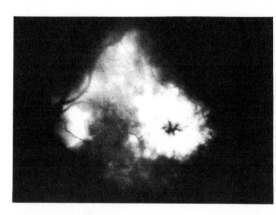

Fig 8.3 Fluorescein angiography demonstrating abnormal leakage of fluorescein around the macula following intraocular surgery. The condition is known as cystoid macular oedema.

also may cause permanent loss of vision, particularly following cataract extraction. Some of the debate about the best cataract operation or implant is directed at the elimination of postoperative cystoid macular oedema. This diagnosis should be considered in patients who have had intraocular surgery, and who have noticed slow visual deterioration in the operated eye.

Retinal detachment

Retinal detachment is the result of the presence of fluid (or occasionally a solid malignant choroidal melanoma or retinoblastoma) between the two layers derived from the primitive retina (*see* Chapter 1 and Plates 1.1, 1.2 and 1.3). These two layers are formed by invagination of the optic vesicle, which is an outgrowth from the forebrain. The outermost of the two layers forms only the pigment epithelium, and part of Bruch's membrane; the inner layer becomes very much thicker and eventually forms the multilayered retina. These two layers are not firmly joined together; indeed we often refer to a 'potential space' between them.

Severe pre-eclamptic toxaemia, malignant hypertension and very low serum protein may be associated with a puddle of 'subretinal'—

intraretinal would be a more accurate term—fluid inferiorly, which absorbs when the diseases resolve. *However, the vast majority of cases of retinal detachment are due to a hole in the retina*; important predisposing factors are myopia, aphakia, increasing age and, less commonly, concussion injury to the eye.

The mechanism of hole formation is important (*see* Plate 8.10). The middle-aged myopic eye begins to develop vitreous degeneration with cavitation and formation of coagula (of the fine fibrils of collagen out of the mucopolysaccharide matrix), which are seen by the patient as a gradually increasing number of 'floating spots' (muscae volitantes). These become particularly obvious when the patient looks at a diffusely bright cloudy sky. This is so common with increasing age, even in the normal eye, as to be regarded as almost physiological. (Such patients can be reassured—with one proviso, below.) The next stage is collapse of the vitreous *with detachment of the vitreous from the retina*. This produces no new symptoms, except perhaps for flashes of light as the vitreous, swirling around because of eye movements, bumps up against the retina. As the vitreous detaches from the retina from behind forwards, the space between the two is filled by fluid which is aqueous humour mixed with some polysaccharide. Unfortunately, particularly in myopes and in the elderly, there are small spots where vitreous is fixed to the retina around the equator (or more anteriorly). Presumably these spots are areas of fibrosis due to some patchy degenerative process in peripheral retina.

The mobile vitreous pulls on one or more of these spots of vitreoretinal ankylosis to produce a retinal hole, or rather a hole in all the layers of retina as far as the pigment epithelium. Through that hole, fluid enters (from behind the detached vitreous) to produce a progressive retinal detachment (or, strictly, an intraretinal separation). This progresses quickly when the hole is in the upper half of the retina—i.e. it often reaches the macular area within a few days. Holes may be round or 'arrowhead' ('horseshoe'), in which latter case the apex points backwards towards the disc. *When the retinal hole is forming, a small retinal blood vessel may be ruptured to discharge a shower of blood into the vitreous cavity, noticed by the patient as a SUDDEN snowstorm or rain-shower.* To the general practitioner or optician, that history within the previous few days is so pathognomonic that the patient should be sent immediately to an ophthalmologist (at least within 24 hours) whether or not vitreous floaters or a retinal hole has been seen. To the ophthalmologist, that history within the previous few days means a very careful search of the *whole* fundus, repeatedly if necessary, with a binocular ophthalmoscope or fundus contact lens (with scleral depression in both cases) to allow the peripheral retina to be seen right out to the ora serrata and beyond. These practices would allow a significant proportion of retinal holes to be found *before* actual retinal detachment occurs: at that stage, cryopexy or light coagulation can be done easily to surround the holes with a mild inflammatory reaction to cause the two layers of the retina to stick together and become permanently organized by fibrous tissue, thus preventing access of fluid to the potential space.

Retinal holes in the lower half of the fundus are much less common, of course. A disinsertion ('dialysis') of peripheral retina may occur inferotemporally, as a result of a developmental defect or, occasionally, an injury. In both these cases the retinal detachment may take months or even years to reach the macula.

As the detachment progresses, usually from above downwards, the patient notices a defect ('black cloud') in his field of vision progressing from below upwards towards the centre. The ophthalmoscopist may see a large black 'mass' superiorly in the fundus, but more usually the layer of subretinal fluid is thin so that the choroidal vasculature is very blurred; 'waves' may be seen in the retina, and both retinal arterioles and venules appear *black*.

Treatment
Treatment is surgical (*see* Plate 8.11 and Fig 8.4). The principles are as follows:

1   A careful examination preoperatively of the *whole* retina will identify all retinal holes.
2   At operation, under direct vision with a binocular ophthalmoscope, the surgeon places a cryoprobe on the surface of the sclera to produce

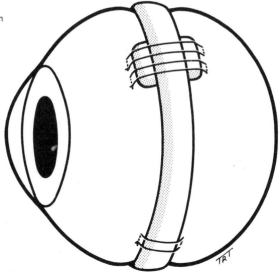

Fig 8.4 Diagram of external view of an eye after operation for retinal detachment. A silicone band encircles and slightly constricts the whole eyeball (to relieve traction by vitreous bands) and aids the localized indentation of a silicone plomb sutured to the surface of the sclera. (*See also* Plate 8.11.)

spots of mild choroiditis around the area to which he judges the hole-bearing areas of retina will return when

3   subretinal fluid is released by a small incision through sclera and choroid, and

4   an encircling silicone band ($\pm$ a silicone plomb over the area of holes) outside the sclera drives the wall of the eyeball (particularly at the hole-bearing areas) towards the retina which otherwise may be rather unwilling to return all the way to the bed it originally left!

5   An intravitreal injection of saline, air or sulphur hexafluoride (SF_6) gas may be given to 'expand' the vitreous cavity and help to drive the retina back into place and close the hole(s). Air or gas are particularly useful in upper half detachments, with the patient sitting up soon after operation.

Step 2 produces a sticky area to hold the retina down until fibrosis occurs during the subsequent few weeks. Step 3 may be omitted if step 4 causes reasonably close approximation of the wall of the eyeball to the retina.

The success rate of operation is around 90% or more, unless unusual circumstances are also present.

Some cases present particular difficulties. Fine fibrous bands may appear in the vitreous and be attached at one or both ends to the retina. These are very common in diabetics, or following vitreous haemorrhages or perforating injuries. When the bands contract, they may pull a hole in the retina *and* hold that area of the retina firmly off its bed. A preliminary cutting of the bands along with vitreous aspiration and fluid replacement—'vitrectomy'—is then required before steps 1 to 5 above are done. Vitrectomy is usually done through a 2 mm diameter hollow metal tube with an oscillating guillotine at its tip, introduced into the vitreous cavity through sclera, choroid and pars plana of retina (i.e. just anterior to the front edge of retina), while a separate finer tube provides fluid infusion.

References

1   Kahn H A, Leibowitz H M, Ganley J P, Kini L M, Colton T, Nickerson R S and Dawber T R. (1977) The eye study. II. Association of ophthalmic pathology with single variables previously measured in the Framingham heart study. *Am J Epidemiol* **106**, 33–41

2   Clayton R M, Cuthbert J, Phillips C I, Bartholomew R S, Stokoe N L, Ffytche T, Reid J McK, Duffy J, Seth J and Alexander M. (1980) Analysis of individual cataract patients and their lenses: a progress report. *Exp Eye Res* **31**, 553–66

3 McKusick V A. (1975) *Mendelian Inheritance in Man,* 5th edn, p. 678. No. 27280. Baltimore and London: Johns Hopkins University Press
4 Fishman G A. (1980) Chloroquine retinopathy. In *Year Book of Ophthalmology,* pp 223–9. Ed. Hughes W F. Chicago: Year Book Medical
5 Mills P V, Beck M and Power B J. (1981) Assessment of the retinal toxicity of hydroxychloroquine. *Trans Ophthalmol Soc UK* **101**, 109–13

9 Neuro-ophthalmology

C I Phillips

One of the great interests of ophthalmology is its involvement in general medicine, particularly neurology. Conversely, for a neurologist or a general physician, neuro-ophthalmology can be an important special interest and indeed a particular knowledge of this subject illuminates many parts of general neurology.

The subject will be considered in anatomical divisions but, within each, only the common or important conditions will be mentioned in order of frequency.

Optic nerve

Disseminated or multiple sclerosis (DS or MS)

This frequently presents with 'retrobulbar neuritis' on one side. Conversely, that condition is almost diagnostic of MS. It presents in the young adult with progressive loss of vision in one eye over a period of 3–7 days until only 'counting fingers' or 'hand movements' vision is present, due to a central scotoma. The cause is a plaque of demyelination in the optic nerve. If the plaque is at the apex of the orbit, where the superior rectus muscle takes origin from the dural sheath of the nerve as well as the nearby frontal bone, pain on looking upwards is characteristic. Very rarely, the plaque may be just behind the cribriform plate at the optic disc, producing 'papillitis' with large splashes of haemorrhage and exudates on the disc which differentiates it from uncomplicated papilloedema (see below); there are very rarely any other causes of 'papillitis'. Visual acuity is very poor in papillitis, but good in papilloedema which is due to raised intracranial pressure.

After 3–5 weeks the visual acuity returns almost completely to normal;

very occasionally it remains poor and a pale disc (primary optic atrophy) ensues. 'Temporal pallor' of the disc is said to be visible after retrobulbar neuritis (RBN) but this is often physiological, especially in myopia.

Provided that there are no other neurological signs or symptoms of MS at the time of RBN, almost 50% of patients will escape any other manifestation of the disease. However, the remainder will develop MS, and around one-third of them will suffer restricted activity by the end of 10 years. I usually feel it is only fair to tell the patient that he has recovered from 'an inflammation of the optic nerve behind the eye', the cause of which is unknown, and that there is a possibility of further attacks of similar inflammation in the same or the other eye or elsewhere in the nervous system (with recovery each time). I advise the patient that for at least four years it is wise to avoid unnecessary stress—for example, pregnancy or ambitious risky career ventures. If he has had no further symptoms in that period, his long-term prognosis is probably better.

Optic atrophy

This, of course, is not a diagnosis. A pale disc, usually with very poor visual acuity, has a large variety of possible causes (including *the* commonest, which is open-angle or chronic simple glaucoma: that disease also produces pathological cupping of the disc—*see* Chapter 5). The next commonest cause in the elderly is a central retinal artery occlusion usually due to a plaque of atheroma at the optic nerve head. The next is occlusion of the blood supply of the optic nerve itself, usually associated with giant cell arteritis and headache, often along with tender temporal arteries (and very commonly a raised ESR). Head injury with or without fractured skull will account for a fair proportion of cases. A few will be due to an intracranial space-occupying lesion, usually with some other signs to suggest a diagnosis.

Papilloedema

Papilloedema is often erroneously suspected when the optic disc merely *appears* to be 'swollen' in a hypermetropic eye. Such an eye is small (*see* Chapters 3 and 4), and the opening in the sclera through which the axes of the ganglion cells pass (optic disc) is also small, hence the crowding of these fibres and an appearance of, or actual, swelling. Haemorrhages do not occur on such a disc, of course. Another pitfall is astigmatism in the patient's eye, which may cause part of the disc margin to *appear* blurred. Indeed any 'optical' cause of blurred vision in the patient (e.g. corneal opacity) may mislead the observer into the diagnosis of blurred disc, for the same reason. The presence of haemorrhages on the disc is an important, but not an essential, part of the diagnosis of papilloedema. A papilloedematous disc can also be seen to be raised above the level of the surrounding fundus, either by parallax or by noting that a different lens in the peep-hole of the ophthalmoscope focuses the apex of the disc when compared with that required for the fundus generally. The disc looks 'juicy' because of the oedema, and its edges become blurred, starting with the nasal side where the blurring remains most marked. Usually the visual acuity is good. The classic cause is an intracranial space-occupying lesion (e.g. a tumour), in which case the papilloedema is usually bilateral though often asymmetrical (and it may be initially unilateral). Papilloedema, headache and vomiting are the triad associated with raised intracranial pressure. Papilloedema is also an important sign of 'malignant hypertension' in need of early treatment but there will also be signs of hypertensive retinopathy elsewhere in the fundus—anyway, the blood pressure will give the diagnosis.

Do not mistake a central retinal vein occlusion (CRVO) for papilloedema, although certainly an eye with CRVO does have papilloedema—but with *widespread* haemorrhages and exudates *all over the fundus (see* Plate 7.2). It is usually unilateral and is accompanied by poor visual acuity of sudden onset.

Pupil reactions

Light reflexes

A normal pupil with normal reactions will contract briskly when a light is shone into the pupil of the same eye ('direct light reaction') and also when the light is shone into the pupil of the other eye ('consensual light reaction'). From these one can deduce that the reflex loop concerned is intact: viz. retina (especially macular area), optic nerve, optic tract to near the lateral geniculate body on the same side, then via a tract of fibres passing medial to the lateral geniculate body to go to *both* right *and* left IIIrd nerve (oculomotor) nuclei in the brain where a relay takes place. Impulses go in a special part of the IIIrd nerve into the orbit and eyeball to stimulate the sphincter muscle of the pupil.

Near reflex

The pathway is different for the reflex contraction of the pupil in response to the stimulation provided by looking at a near object—the 'near' reflex, associated with accommodation and convergence. As before, retina (especially macula) and optic nerve are involved but the afferent nerves actually enter the lateral geniculate body. After relay in the lateral geniculate body, impulses go on to the occipital cortex from which a relay passes (?)via cortical association fibres to the 'frontomotor eye field' in the frontal cortex (posteriorly) and then to the IIIrd nerve nucleus (relay) and then into the IIIrd nerve to reach the sphincter muscle of the pupil (producing miosis) as well as the ciliary muscle (for accommodation) and medial rectus (for convergence).

Abnormal reactions

Probably the commonest cause of abnormal pupil reflexes is the result of atropine, or tropicamide or cyclopentolate eyedrops used to dilate the pupil. When their action is maximal, no response of the pupil can be elicited. Their effect passes off in 7 days, 6 hours and 24 hours respectively. Similarly, pilocarpine, physostigmine (eserine) and di-isopropyl-fluorophosphonate (DFP) constrict the pupil maximally, which prevents any additional response to light or for near.

In an eye clinic, probably the commonest numerical causes of abnormal pupil shape *and* reactions are local lesions in the iris or pupil—for example, perforating injuries (including operations!) and iridocyclitis which have mechanically distorted irises and pupils and have fixed them to lens or lens remnants or vitreous by fibrous tissue or inflammatory exudate.

Another common-sense situation relates to blindness. If one eye only is totally blind from, say, chronic simple glaucoma or pressure of a tumour on one optic nerve, no direct reaction to light is possible and of course the absence of an afferent pathway from that eye prevents a consensual reaction in the other normal one. However, when a light is shone into the normal eye, a good consensual reaction in the blind eye will occur because the efferent pathways to that eye are intact. Similarly, the pupil in such a blind eye, if the other is normal, will contract in response to close work.

Myotonic (= Holmes–Adie's or Adie's) pupil

This usually presents in a girl in her late teens who has noticed one pupil dilated for a few weeks. Check that there is no risk of any drugs' having entered that eye. There is also blurred vision for close work in that eye because of paresis of accommodation. Characteristically the pupil contracts very slowly to a sustained stimulus from light, directly and consensually, but contracts briskly for near. A variant has a quick light reaction and a slow near reaction. Sometimes the condition is bilateral. There is often absence of the ankle and knee jerks. The cause of this very odd disease is unknown but pathological changes have been observed in the ciliary ganglion in the orbit. Surprisingly, the syndrome carries no implication of serious CNS or other disease later.

The Argyll Robertson pupil

This is rarely seen nowadays, because tertiary syphilis of which it is typical is uncommon. There is complete absence of a response to light, directly and consensually, but a brisk response for near. It is usually associated with absence of the knee and ankle jerks. These similarities to Adie's syndrome are quite superficial because other properties make the differentiation easy: *Argyll Robertson pupils are invariably bilateral, very small and irregular in shape.* Men aged 40 and over are those usually affected.

Chiasmal lesions

It is quite remarkably interesting and important that the axons from the ganglion cells of the nasal half of the *right* retina *and* the nasal half of the *left* retina cross to the opposite side at the chiasma. But the axons from the ganglion cells of the temporal half of the *right* and the temporal half of the *left* retina remain on the same side (Fig 9.1). The precise but invisible

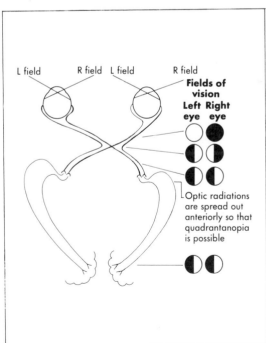

L field R field L field R field
Fields of vision
Left Right eye eye

Optic radiations are spread out anteriorly so that quadrantanopia is possible

Fig 9.1 Diagram of a horizontal section through the brain at the level of the eyes shows the optic sensory pathways to the occipital or visual cortex. The anterior limits of the retinae are indicated . This allows a wide visual field. A lesion of the right optic nerve causes blindness in the right eye with no effect on the left field. A midline chiasmal lesion causes bitemporal hemianopia. A lesion of the optic tract or occipital cortex produces a contralateral hemianopia, with a sharp edge. An irregular-edged though homonymous defect in the contralateral field results from a lesion in the optic radiations because they spread out as they circumvent the inferior horn of the lateral ventricle; more or less than a quadrantanopia may be found.

dividing line in the retina between 'nasal' and 'temporal' is a vertical one through the fovea. ('Chiasma' is derived from a Greek word which has the sound 'ch' as in the Scottish 'loch' but a symbol like the English 'X'.) One exception to this arrangement exists in albino animals and humans, in all of whom some axons from retinal ganglion cells temporal to the normal vertical retinal dividing line cross at the chiasma to the other side.

A bitemporal hemianopia must mean a midline lesion of the chiasma, usually due to an enlargement of the pituitary gland (eosinophil adenoma in acromegaly or chromophobe adenoma) in an adult; in a child a suprasellar cyst may cause it. These lesions may extend forwards or backwards towards one side to cause complete blindness on that side; in the other eye, only the temporal loss is still present.

Post-chiasmal lesions

A lesion affecting the *right* optic *tract* behind the chiasma (*see* Fig 9.1) will produce a homonymous hemianopia on the left side—i.e. the left half of the field of the left eye *and* the left half of the field of the right eye will be lost. This is usually a total loss of all sight within the half-field because the tracts have a small cross-section. After the relay in the lateral geniculate body, the optic radiations are spread out as they arch inferotemporally anterior to the inferior horn of the lateral ventricle *en route* to the occipital cortex where they occupy a considerable surface area around the calcarine fissure. Accordingly, lesions along that part of the pathway are seldom large enough to destroy all the fibres and so only, say, a quadrant of the field on the opposite side is missing: the area of field loss in the two eyes is identical ('congruous'). Tumours of the temporal lobe, and vascular lesions anywhere along the post-geniculate pathway, are the usual causes of congruous loss of part of the contralateral half-field.

Sudden complete loss of all vision in both eyes, *with retention of the pupillary light reflexes, direct and consensual,* is usually explained by a blockage in the basilar artery (atherothrombotic) at its upper end because it bifurcates there into the right and left posterior cerebral arteries. Surprisingly, there is usually no other neurological defect apart from blindness, and indeed the patient may be less aware of his state than when his blindness is due to, say, bilateral blockage of the arterial supply to his optic nerve as in giant cell arteritis.

Another useful clinical point is that a hemiplegic patient may also have a hemianopia which he may not realize. It is probably due to the proximity of the optic pathway to the pyramidal pathway. A few seconds' testing of each visual field in all four quadrants (to finger movements) is well worth while in many patients with possibly related symptoms—the patient can seldom describe exactly a homonymous hemianopia. A homonymous hemianopia may also accompany alexia (inability to recognize letters) or nominal aphasia (inability to name an object though aware of its function—e.g. a pen held in front of the patient): these are due to impaired function of the parieto-occipital cortex just anterior to the occipital cortex of the left side in right-handed people.

Diplopia and extraocular muscle paralysis

History taking

Frequently a patient complains of 'double vision' when in fact 'blurred vision' would be a more appropriate description. Accordingly, very early in the history, the questions must be asked, 'Does the double vision disappear if you shut the left eye?' and then, 'Does the double vision disappear if you shut the right eye?' In cases of misalignment of the two visual axes (e.g. due to weakness of an extraocular muscle) the answers to both questions will be 'yes'—the diplopia is binocular; that is, present only when *both* eyes are open and it disappears when either eye is shut. If the so-called diplopia is really due to blurred vision in one eye, or in each eye separately, the 'diplopia' will *remain* when the right and/or the left eye is shut: this can be confirmed by checking with the patient—'does the double vision *remain* when you shut the left eye' and '. . . right . . .'. Such blurred vision in one eye or in each eye separately is usually found in the elderly and is due to cataract, but other causes are astigmatism, myopia and corneal opacities.

Diagnostic strategy

When the examiner is sure that binocular diplopia is the problem, and the diagnosis is not immediately obvious (e.g. recent faciomaxillary fractures, proptosis), a good plan is to consider possible causes systematically from anterior to posterior in the following order:

1   Orbital lesions, often interfering mechanically with ocular movements. Dysthyroid orbital lesions are the commonest (infiltration of muscles and fat with lymphocytes followed by fibrosis), then trauma to the orbit. Neoplasms, primary or secondary (locally from sinuses, pharynx etc. or blood-borne metastasis), are occasional culprits; do not forget the lacrimal gland.

2   Neuromuscular junction. In myasthenia gravis, the onset may be quite sudden and remarkably selective of one or few extraocular

muscles: surprisingly often only one eye or eyelid is affected. A Tensilon test is usually positive.

3 Muscular lesions. Selective dystrophies of the extraocular muscles, excluding the general musculature, sometimes occur, but usually cause symmetrical reduction in ocular movements in all directions of gaze without diplopia. The levator palpebrae superioris may be the only one affected, producing bilateral symmetrical ptosis of the upper lids. (*See also* item 1, above.)

4 Nerve lesions usually produce only weakness of movement of the eyeball, which is difficult for the examiner to detect when he asks the patient to watch his finger about 1 metre in front of the patient as he moves it to the right then to the left, then up and (holding the upper lids up) down and to the intermediate positions. The student should see the orthoptist identifying the weak muscle by the Lees or Hess screen.

Complete paralysis of an extraocular muscle is seldom present. A diagnosis of, say, a complete left lateral rectus paralysis (due to a complete lesion of the left abducent nerve) is easy when the observer notes that the left eye cannot move beyond the mid-point when the patient looks to his left. The patient notices increasingly wide horizontal separation of diplopic images as he looks to the left.

Nerve weakness with diplopia but without obvious impairment of a movement is more common. Questioning can usually identify the affected muscle. Horizontal diplopia only, greater to left or right, is more likely to be due to impaired function of the left or right lateral rectus muscle respectively than a right or left medial rectus respectively: the reason is that the former are supplied by a single nerve (abducent) whereas the latter share the oculomotor nerve, a lesion of which would also affect other muscles to produce a vertical separation with or without tilt (*see* below).

A purely vertical diplopia *without* a significant tilt of the images is probably due to a lesion of one superior or inferior ('vertical') rectus muscle. If the separation of images increases on looking upwards, a superior rectus is affected: cover one eye to eliminate one image; the eye responsible for the image further away from centre has the weak muscle. If the separation increases on downward gaze, an inferior rectus is affected: covering one eye will eliminate one image; the eye with the further-away image has the weak muscle. Either situation is more likely to be due to a lesion in the orbit (e.g. dysthyroid myopathy) than a lesion of the oculomotor nerve, since only a small part of the nerve would have to be involved to explain it on a neurological basis.

A significant *tilt* of the more peripheral image (often with a small vertical separation) suggests weakness of an oblique muscle. Again, the superior oblique is more likely to be the culprit than the inferior oblique because a selective lesion of only part of the oculomotor nerve (supplying the inferior oblique) is less likely than a lesion affecting the whole of the trochlear nerve (which supplies only the superior oblique muscle). In a trochlear nerve paresis the vertical separation is maximized when the affected eye is turned towards the nose as well as downwards, and again the more peripheral image (found by covering one eye) belongs to the paretic eye.

The ophthalmologist often resorts to the Hess or Lees screen to identify the weak muscle.

To consider the problem even more generally, a young adult with recent diplopia without any other symptoms probably has multiple sclerosis and his symptoms should disappear in 3–6 weeks. An elderly person with recent diplopia and no other symptoms probably has a vascular lesion of (part of) a cranial nerve which may not recover. A primary or secondary intracranial tumour should be considered as a rare possibility in the differential diagnosis in both cases. The sudden onset of diplopia and headache would suggest an intracranial aneurysm at any age.

An *internuclear ophthalmoplegia* is an interesting exercise in applied anatomy. In the young it is usually due to multiple sclerosis (and recovers in a few weeks) and in the elderly to a very localized vascular lesion. Suppose the anterior end of the left medial longitudinal fasciculus is affected. When the examiner's finger (at which the patient has been asked to look) moves to the right, efferent impulses will start from the right frontomotor eye field of the cortex. Some are destined for the part of the left IIIrd nucleus serving the left medial rectus muscle, but will be interrupted in the left medial longitudinal fasciculus and so the left eye will fail to turn to the right; others will succeed in reaching the right VIth (abducent) nucleus, and so the right eye will be turned to the right—with nystagmoid jerks as the cortex (probably) tries to reinforce the stimuli to the unresponsive left medial rectus muscle. This is called 'ataxic nystagmus'.

Headache

Patients with headaches are often wrongly referred to an optician or ophthalmologist because of a traditional and usually erroneous belief that refractive errors cause headaches and that treatment with spectacles will cure them. A careful history of original time of onset, duration of individual headaches, frequency, quality and site of pain/discomfort, precipitating causes and whether relieved by analgesics will usually show quite clearly the impossiblity of a diagnosis of refractive error as a cause. Perhaps one exception is the hypermetrope or early presbyope who may have aching eyes and some frontal headache after 15 minutes' close work, relieved by stopping reading and restarted when close work is resumed.

Of course, headache around an eye with acute closed-angle glaucoma or a corneal ulcer will be expected but usually not mentioned, and certainly would be very, very rarely a presenting symptom.

The causes of headaches erroneously referred are several. *Trigeminal neuralgia* occurs in elderly patients who complain of very sudden attacks of *severe* pain in or behind one eye and *lasting a few seconds*: at first they may occur only once in several weeks, but over a period of a year or two the attacks often increase in frequency to several times daily. When the maxillary division of the Vth cranial nerve is affected, the ENT department may receive the patient; when the mandibular division is involved, the dentist may be the first resort.

Frontal sinusitis usually starts only a few weeks before the patient reaches the ophthalmologist: the right or left low frontal pain occurs daily, starting at, say, 11.00 am, and reaches a plateau during an hour or so, and remains until bed-time, to disappear by the following morning. The cycle repeats itself daily. Pressure upwards by the examiner's thumb just behind the nasal end of the supraorbital margin will elicit tenderness on the affected side.

It is vitally important for general practitioners, physicians and neurologists as well as ophthalmologists to diagnose the headache of *giant cell arteritis* as early as possible because it may be complicated by sudden loss of vision in one eye, *and at any time thereafter in the other eye* (i.e. total bilateral blindness) due to an arteritic blockage to the blood supply of the optic disc—'ischaemic optic neuropathy'. The headache is constant, distributed diffusely over the vertex and reduced by analgesics; there is usually, but not necessarily, pain in, or tenderness of, a temporal artery—a previous name for the disease was 'temporal arteritis'. The patient has general malaise. Duration may be weeks or months.

The ophthalmologist usually sees the patient following sudden blindness in one eye—and he has learned to consider giant cell arteritis as a possible cause in all such cases. There is usually a history of headache, of course, and a markedly raised ESR. It is a tragedy if the patient loses the sight in the second eye while waiting for an appointment to the ophthalmologist about the sudden blindness in the first eye: the general practitioner should do an urgent ESR in all cases of sudden blindness in one eye due to arterial block (not in venous thrombosis, vitreous haemorrhage, etc.). A biopsy of one temporal artery usually provides histological confirmation of a diagnosis, but systemic steroids in high dosage initially should be given urgently on the basis of clinical findings and the ESR—i.e. biopsy is unnecessary in the vast majority of cases.

Migraine ('idiopathic') is a major reason for unnecessary spectacles! Again the history is usually typical—a late teenager has a right or left frontal headache for a few hours once in a few weeks, often preceded by flashing lights in one or other half-field or in the central area of the field, and often followed after an hour or so by nausea with or without vomiting. A first-degree relative is often similarly affected. Another feature which quells anxiety in the physician who is always worried about missing an aneurysm or intracranial tumour is that the headache or visual disturbance affects sometimes one side and sometimes the other, or both simultaneously.

Special neurological investigations

This chapter has been restricted to a limited range of clinical neuro-ophthalmology, and has excluded deeper investigations which are the province of the specialist neurologist and neurosurgeon.

However, a recent advance in imaging techniques applied to medicine is of considerable interest: nuclear magnetic resonance. It is even less invasive than the CAT scan because it does not involve ionizing radiation, and no adverse effects have so far been reported. It has particular application in neurological diseases, and also in orbital conditions (*see* Chapter 13).

The whole patient, or the part to be examined, is placed within a uniform static magnetic field: protons in the chemical nuclei of his tissues behave like tiny bar magnets and align themselves in the field. By means of a coil surrounding the patient, additional magnetic pulses (electromagnetic waves of radiofrequency) are applied which very briefly rotate the nuclei: the time taken for the nuclei to 'relax' back to their previous position depends on the interaction of their protons with each other, and with surrounding nuclei and molecules. As the magnetization due to 'relaxation' changes, it induces an electrical signal in a receiver coil which surrounds the patient; those signals are converted by a computer (within seconds) into a picture on a colour video screen. It looks superficially rather similar to a CAT scan.

Vascular and Diabetic Retinopathies

D B Archer

Introduction

The transparent ocular media present the physician with an unrivalled opportunity to study a major vascular system of the body *in vivo*. Optical instruments now permit direct observation of the smallest retinal vessels. This can provide valuable clues to the patient's systemic vascular state.

Examination and diagnostic methods

Direct ophthalmoscopy

Evaluation of the retinal vasculature is best done after full dilatation of the pupil (0.5 or 1.0% tropicamide or 0.5 or 1.0% cyclopentolate hydrochloride with or without 10% phenylephrine eyedrops). The retinal vessels can be seen by either direct or indirect illumination, and some appreciation of depth can be gained by parallax (i.e. the observer moving his eye plus ophthalmoscope across the pupillary aperture). With good illumination, direct ophthalmoscopy will allow the smallest arterioles and venules (20 μm in diameter) to be seen. In young patients, it is even possible to identify the individual capillaries of the perifoveal capillary network (5–15 μm). Red-free light (green filter) may improve resolution by converting the retinal vessels to black and the fundus to green. Abnormalities should be recorded on a simple diagram.

    Exaggerated venous pulsation at the optic disc may indicate raised intraocular pressure or cardiovascular disease (e.g. aortic incompetence). *Spontaneous venous pulsation is a reliable indicator that intracranial pressure is normal, but its absence is not a dependable guide to raised intracranial pressure.*

Indirect ophthalmoscopy

The retinal vasculature may also be examined using this more specialized technique. It provides a stereoscopic view of the ocular fundus at a smaller magnification than direct ophthalmoscopy and is particularly valuable in seeing fundus lesions in spite of lens or vitreous opacities.

Slit-lamp fundus microscopy

This can be adapted to combine many of the advantages of direct and indirect ophthalmoscopy—i.e. bright illumination, high magnification of the fundus, stereopsis and an erect image. A contact lens is used to eliminate the curvature and refractive power of the cornea, and the fundus is then directly viewed using a slit-lamp microscope.

Ophthalmodynamometry

The central retinal artery blood pressure can be measured by the technique of ophthalmodynamometry. The intraocular pressure is raised by the application of an external force to the eye, and the point at which arterial pulsation is first detected in the central retinal vessels is taken as the diastolic pressure of the central retinal artery. The point at which arterial pulsation just ceases is a measure of systolic pressure. This technique may help in identifying patients with severe unilateral carotid artery obstruction, but great accuracy is impossible.

Fundus photography

This is indispensible for the accurate documentation of the natural course of various disease processes—particularly retinal tumours, diabetic retinopathy, macular oedema and retinal neovascularization. Stereoscopic fundus photography helps locate the level of the abnormality within the retina.

Fluorescein angiography

The retinal vessels are vividly outlined by means of the non-toxic fluorescent dye, sodium fluorescein. About 5 ml of a dilute solution is injected into an arm vein and quickly reaches the retinal vasculature. The dye absorbs light from the ophthalmoscope or the fundus camera, but emits light of a different wavelength. Only that emitted light is allowed to reach the observer (or the film in the camera) by means of barrier filters in the system which excludes all other wavelengths. In most cases the fundus camera has to be used to obtain a series of photographic recordings during the few seconds of passage of the dye through the retinal arteries and veins. This technique accurately assesses retinal vascular haemodynamics and identifies subtle structural abnormalities of the retinal microvasculature. Normal retinal vessels (like cerebral vessels) do not leak fluorescein, so this technique is a sensitive measure of vascular competence. The patient should be warned that the renal vessels do leak fluorescein!

Fluorescein angiography also gives important information about the choroidal and papillary circulations and the retinal pigment epithelium.

Basic responses of the retinal vasculature to stress and disease

The retinal vasculature is one of the most organized and specialized networks of blood vessels in the body. It provides the retina with a blood flow considerably in excess of most tissues and has a high capillary pressure which serves to offset the opposing intraocular pressure (10–21 mmHg). By virtue of its tightly adherent and relatively impermeable endothelial cells, the vessels regulate fluid transport between the intravascular and extravascular compartments of the retina and so stabilize its internal environment. The retinal vessels autoregulate despite significant variations in intraocular pressure to maintain nutrition of the retina.

Alterations in vascular calibre

Alterations in vascular calibre are a response to various factors. Retinal arteries dilate in the presence of hypoxia (pulseless disease), in certain hyperdynamic circulatory states (thyroid disease) and secondary to focal degenerative processes (e.g. arteriosclerotic macroaneurysms). Venous dilatation results from reduced oxygen tension in the blood (cyanotic heart disease) or venous obstruction, and is very characteristic of early diabetic retinopathy.

Arterial and arteriolar constriction is a response to increased intraluminar pressure—i.e. hypertension (unless prevented by arteriosclerosis)—and is also a response to widespread retinal atrophy (retinitis pigmentosa). The immature retinal circulation of the prematurely born infant responds to high concentrations of oxygen by constriction, with the risk of subsequent blindness when 'retrolental fibroplasia' may develop (see Chapter 1).

Alterations in vascular permeability

Changes in vascular permeability, particularly of the endothelium, usually cause the following conditions.

Retinal oedema
This results from the accumulation of fluid, molecules and ions in the extracellular compartments. Incompetence of the superficial (arterial) retinal capillaries (e.g. in accelerated hypertension) leads to *inner* retinal oedema; nerve fibres are separated and so appear as glistening and opalescent streaks. As oedema subsides, 'hard' exudates (lipid and protein) accumulate and often become distributed in a radial fashion about the fovea (macular star) or the optic disc. Oedema of the optic disc (e.g. papilloedema or papillitis) is often accompanied by some oedema of the immediately surrounding retina.

Retinal venous disease typically produces oedema in the *outer* plexiform layer of the retina. Macular oedema may occur in uveitis, or following cataract extraction or after obstruction of the tributary vein near the macula. It often leads eventually to the formation of multiloculated cyst-like spaces which give a characteristic petaloid pattern—i.e. like the petals of a flower—on fluorescein angiography (microcystoid oedema).

Retinal exudates
Retinal exudates are of two main kinds:

1 *Hard (fatty) exudates* are round, discrete, yellow–white lesions located within the outer plexiform layer of the retina. They may form a star-like (stellate) or a circular (circinate) pattern depending on their location within the retina and the sites of greatest vascular incompetence. Histologically, they consist of altered blood constituents and retinal macrophages; as vascular competence is recovered they become more discrete and often disappear. If vascular incompetence is prolonged, hard exudates aggregate and cause irreversible changes in the retinal receptors with loss of vision.
2 *Soft exudates* ('cotton wool spots') are foci of inner retinal ischaemia, generally indicating retinal arteriolar occlusion (see later).

Retinal haemorrhages
Retinal haemorrhages may result from raised intraluminar pressure (vein occlusion), degenerative changes within the vessel wall (macroaneurysm)

or neovascularization (a response to ischaemia). They are usually classified descriptively as follows.

1   *Superficial retinal haemorrhages* (*flame-shaped, striate*) arise from the inner retinal or circumpapillary capillary beds. They are distributed along the nerve fibre layer and vary from small splinter haemorrhages (striate), as in hypertension, to large fan- or flame-shaped haemorrhages several disc diameters in size, which occur in diabetes and leukaemia.

2   *Deep retinal haemorrhages* are located in the outer plexiform layers. Their vertical and horizontal dimensions are limited by the glial fibres of Mueller, so they tend to be small, circular and discrete (dot and blot haemorrhages). They usually disappear slowly (without complications) because of their small surface area.

3   *Subretinal haemorrhages* usually originate from fragile new vessels which have grown from the choroid in senile macular degeneration to lie beneath the retinal pigment epithelium, or between it and the inner layer of retina. These haemorrhages tend to occur in the macular region, and damage rods and cones in that area, producing a central scotoma. They may be bright red, deep red or black, depending on their density and location. They absorb slowly, often with proliferation of the retinal pigment epithelium, scar formation and loss of vision. Haemorrhages under the retinal pigment epithelium are often due to tears in the choroid (produced, for example, by concussive injuries to the anterior eyeball, by a contre-coup mechanism as in concussion injuries to the brain) as well as due to senile macular degeneration mentioned above. They appear as large, dark grey mounds due to the superimposed colour of the retinal pigment epithelium and may be mistaken for choroidal naevi or small malignant melanomata.

4   *White centre haemorrhages* (Roth spots) are due to focal accumulations of white cells at the centre of large haemorrhages and occur mainly in leukaemia, aplastic anaemia and Wernicke's encephalopathy.

5   *Preretinal haemorrhage* is a pool of blood at the posterior pole, trapped between the internal limiting membrane of the retina and the posterior vitreous face. Within an hour or so after the sudden loss of vision it produces, the red cells sediment to leave a horizontal fluid level. The cause is sudden back-pressure on the retinal veins, especially due to a sudden rise in intracranial pressure in subarachnoid haemorrhage (traumatic or 'spontaneous'); ophthalmoscopy can provide a useful diagnostic clue in the suddenly unconscious patient. **Do not use a mydriatic in these cases:** the neurosurgeon needs to

observe the state of dilatation of the pupils to monitor progress—
'coning' will cause pressure on the IIIrd cranial nerve at the
tentorium, hence unilateral (later bilateral) dilatation of the pupils.

Vitreous haemorrhages
These may originate from the retinal, papillary or, more rarely, the
choroidal circulation. They are typically caused by trauma, retinal and
papillary neovascularization (especially in diabetes mellitus) and
'spontaneous' retinal tears. The patient notices a sudden snowstorm of
floaters, or a 'film of smoke', before the eye. If a retinal tear is present,
flashes of light may accompany or precede the vitreous haemorrhage,
either because vitreoretinal adhesions pull on the retina or because mobile
detached vitreous strikes the retina; mechanical stimulation of retina can
produce a sensation of light (*see* Chapter 8 and Plates 8.10 and 8.11).
Minor vitreous haemorrhages usually resolve rapidly, but severe
haemorrhages may persist for months or years. Vitrectomy may be
effective in clearing long-standing dense haemorrhages and achieves most
success where macular function is preserved.

Structural changes in the vessel walls

The walls of normal retinal vessels are transparent. The layer of plasma
which constitutes the peripheral portion of the blood stream is also
transparent. Therefore, during ophthalmoscopy only the central red cell
column is visible in a normal vessel. Changes in the character or structure
of the vessel wall modify the visibility or alter the hue of the red cell
column and so can provide important clues about local and systemic
vascular disease.

Sclerosis
Arteriosclerosis is common and associated with an increased collagen
content of the vessel wall. (Atheroma has only occasionally been
described in the central retinal artery.) In early disease and ageing the
light reflex that normally occupies the centre of the blood column is
widened, and white lines may become obvious at the sides of the arteries.
In advanced disease, the arterial wall becomes opaque and obscures the
red cell column to varying degrees. Severely involved vessels often have
parallel yellow–white segments along their course ('sheathing').
Occasionally the vessel lumen is totally obscured ('ghost vessels')—e.g.
vein occlusion or old retrolental fibroplasia.

In the elderly, small areas of advanced retinal arteriosclerosis are often
found in the retinal periphery (lattice degeneration): the occluded vessels
appear as white criss-crossing lines, and the nearby retina is typically

atrophic. Full-thickness retinal holes occur in about 18% of cases, and may lead to retinal detachment.

Phlebosclerosis is usually secondary to occlusive vascular disease, and is first apparent as subtle fine white lines along the peripheral blood column. In severe disease the vessel wall may become completely white although fluorescein angiography may still confirm some circulation.

Retinal periphlebitis (Eales' disease) is a very distinctive and fascinating clinical entity of unknown cause (?allergy to tuberculoprotein). It affects young males, especially in India, but is rare in Western countries. The venules in the *peripheral* retina typically show, at first, many patches of inflammatory thickening which obscures the red cell column. Nearby retina is oedematous and some inflammatory cells wander into nearby vitreous. Recurrent vitreous haemorrhages occur and blindness often ensues, although some control can be achieved with local laser treatment and systemic steroids. Differential diagnosis includes sickle cell disease.

(An insignificant patchy periphlebitis may also occur in multiple sclerosis and in inflammatory diseases of the retina which involves retinal blood vessels—e.g. toxoplasmosis, pars planitis and sarcoidosis.)

Collaterals

Collaterals link obstructed and non-obstructed vessels—e.g. in vein occlusion. They have an irregular meandering course, and are usually patent and competent (on fluorescein angiography).

Arteriovenous crossing changes

These occur because retinal arteries and veins share a common adventitial coat at the point of crossing. As the arterial wall becomes thicker with age or arteriosclerosis, the blood column in the vein becomes obscured and eventually narrowed ('nipping') to some degree. Increasing pressure by the artery dilates the vein slightly peripheral to the pressure point. Straightening of the arteries in hypertension with or without arteriosclerosis deflects the vein peripherally and alters the angle of crossing.

Microaneurysms

Microaneurysms comprise one of the commonest responses of the retinal microvasculature to disease and can be identified by ophthalmoscopy, slit-lamp biomicroscopy or fluorescein angiography. They are seen as small red dots (25–100 μm in diameter) and are present most typically in diabetes but also, to a smaller extent, in hypertension, sickle cell disease, vein occlusion, glaucoma, dysproteinaemias and in the ageing retina. In diabetes they predominantly occur at the posterior pole of the eye, whereas in branch retinal vein obstruction they are located within the distribution of the obstructed vein. Fluorescein angiography confirms that there are always many more microaneurysms present than those identified by ophthalmoscopy. Most microaneurysms are symptomless, but when multiple and incompetent they may be associated with intraretinal oedema and hard exudates.

Macroaneurysms

Macroaneurysms typically arise from arteriosclerotic retinal arteries or arterioles and affect elderly hypertensive individuals. Large arterial aneurysms also occur in Coats' disease, in Leber's miliary aneurysms and in retinal angiomatosis. Most macroaneurysms are symptomless although some perimacular aneurysms may lead to chronic fluid accumulation, cystoid macular oedema or haemorrhage.

Intraretinal microvascular abnormalities ('hairpin capillaries')

These are abnormal dilated channels within the retina, and occur in a wide variety of diseases characterized by stasis and ischaemia—for example, diabetes, branch vein occlusion and sickle cell retinopathy. Some probably represent attempts at intraretinal repair and neovascularization, and are best identified by fluorescein angiography.

Tears and ruptures

Tears and ruptures of retinal blood vessels may be produced by severe contusional or perforating eye injuries. Compressive chest injuries may cause rupture of small unsupported retinal venules. '*Spontaneous*' retinal tears, also involving blood vessels, are associated with detachment of the posterior vitreous face, especially in high myopia. It is a good axiom that 'spontaneous' vitreous haemorrhage in the absence of established retinopathy should be considered due to a retinal tear until proven otherwise and a meticulous search of the retinal periphery with scleral depression undertaken to find a retinal hole or tear with or without incipient retinal detachment (*see* Chapter 8 and Plates 8.10 and 8.11).

Vascular obstruction and occlusion

Occlusion of the central retinal artery

Such occlusion (due to atheroma at the optic disc in most cases) usually produces a complete infarct of the retina, except for the layer of rods and cones because that is nourished by diffusion of oxygen and nutrients from the choroid. Embolus is a less common cause; for example, blood clot from a mural thrombus in the heart or platelet emboli from an ulcerating atheromatous plaque at the origin of the internal carotid artery. Emboli typically cause transient loss of vision for a few seconds ('amaurosis fugax'), before disimpacting and migrating to more peripheral retinal arterioles where they may be visible as yellow or white spots, Fibrin and other plasma constituents may seal the collapsed vessels downstream of the obstruction but, in any case, there is little chance of significant collateral formation because the retinal vasculature is an end-artery system.

Cells of the infarcted retina degenerate and swell (intracellular oedema) and so become white and opaque to the ophthalmoscopist. The retina, like the brain, has little extracellular space, so there is little opportunity for extracellular oedema. This is most striking where the retina is thickest—i.e. at the posterior pole, surrounding the fovea centralis (*see* Chapter 1 and Figs 1.1 and 1.2). In contrast, the very thin, transparent fovea remains bright red in colour because choroidal circulation is visible through it (*see* Fig 1.2 and Plate 10.8). Most fluid absorbs within two or three weeks, so the retina will appear remarkably normal apart from attenuated retinal arteries and arterioles.

Precapillary arteriolar occlusion

Cotton wool spots or soft exudates are discrete, opaque swellings of the inner retina that occur in severe systemic vascular disorders characterized by arteriolar occlusion; e.g. diabetes, accelerated hypertension, toxaemia of pregnancy, systemic lupus erythematosus and retinal microemboli. Histologically they are the distended stumps of the axons of ganglion cells, which appear white because of the light-scattering properties of the accumulated organelles (e.g. mitochondria) within the distended terminals. Cotton wool spots may develop from any injury to the nerve fibre layer of the retina, leading to gross stasis of orthograde or retrograde axoplasmic transport in ganglion cell axons.

Cotton wool spots measure about one-third of a disc diameter and are typically confined to the posterior fundus. Fresh cotton wool spots have a striking grey/white appearance with ill-defined borders and are located within the nerve fibre layer. They appear rapidly, often being noted within a few hours of an acute ischaemic episode, and then gradually fade, becoming grey and fragmenting before becoming fully absorbed in about six weeks.

Fluorescein angiography shows that most cotton wool spots are non-fluorescent and that the non-perfused capillary bed is typically surrounded by clusters of microaneurysms and dilated capillaries.

Larger areas of ischaemic retina are common in diabetics and have a light grey rather than a white colour, perhaps due to the fact that they have developed chronically and there is no acute accumulation of axoplasmic debris.

Central retinal and tributary venous occlusion ('thrombotic glaucoma')
Occlusion of the central retinal vein (CRVO), or of one of its tributaries, is usually due to atheroma or severe arteriosclerosis of the central retinal artery, or a branch of it, where the artery and vein are in contact or cross. The raised and fluctuating intraocular pressure in glaucoma is sometimes a precipitating factor. The whole retina, or a segment, shows large numbers of flame-shaped haemorrhages (because of rupture of venules from back-pressure) with numerous soft exudates. In CRVO the disc may be obscured by haemorrhages or disc oedema.* (In contrast, papilloedema due to raised intracranial pressure is restricted to the disc where *small* haemorrhages—few or multiple—usually occur; there are no widespread *retinal* haemorrhages.)

Central retinal vein occlusion causes severe permanent loss of vision. Tributary vein occlusion will produce a loss of field of vision corresponding to the affected area unless the haemorrhages involve the macula, in which case there is loss of central vision.

Because of the diffusion from ischaemic (but not completely infarcted) retina of a substance (or substances) which stimulates neovasculogenesis, new vessels often appear in the iris and in the angle of the anterior chamber. The trabecular meshwork is also affected resulting in a severe 'thrombotic glaucoma' about three months after the CRVO in about 30% of cases. To prevent this disastrous outcome, often requiring enucleation because of severe pain, the ischaemic retina can be converted to dead tissue by widespread photocoagulation.

Retinal and papillary neovascularization
As a response to ischaemia, the retinal vasculature has the ability to elaborate new vessels. As mentioned above, the stimulus is probably chemical. The process is generally slow and incomplete and may be without consequence for central visual function.

Preretinal new vessels appear to originate from the venous side of the circulation, and gain access to the preretinal region through defects in the internal limiting membrane which typically occur in the immediate vicinity of large retinal veins. New retinal vessels typically complicate a disease process characterized by extensive inner retinal ischaemia; e.g. diabetes, large order vein occlusion, sickle cell disease and retrolental fibroplasia. The new vessels ramify between the internal limiting membrane and the posterior vitreous face. They preferentially attach themselves to the posterior vitreous face and when this membrane detaches there is forward movement of the new vessels often associated with rupture and haemorrhage. Fibrous tissue typically develops

---

* In this chapter the term 'papilloedema' is used only when disc swelling is due to raised intracranial pressure.

alongside new vessels and, if profuse, may cause retinal corrugations, traction detachment and partial or full-thickness retinal holes. New vessels may also sprout from the disc directly into the vitreous body.

Specific retinal vascular diseases and syndromes: retinal vascular stasis, obstruction and occlusion

Aortic–carotid artery insufficiency

The blood supply to the eye and retinal circulation may be affected by obstruction or occlusion of blood vessels carrying blood between the heart and the eye.

Pulseless disease. This condition results from stenosis of the major branches of the aorta—i.e. the carotid, brachiocephalic, subclavian and vertebral branches. Pulses become weak or absent and patients may suffer varying degrees of cerebrovascular ischaemia. Atheromatous deposits are the commonest cause of pulseless disease, although diffuse arteritis of unknown aetiology (Takayasu's disease), giant cell arteritis or syphilis may also cause severe stenosis. When blood flow to the eye is significantly reduced, transient loss of vision (amaurosis fugax), visual obscurations or sudden blindness may occur. The peripheral retinal circulation typically shows evidence of stasis and collapse, often associated with formation of arteriovenous anastomoses in areas of non-perfusion. Severe ischaemia may precipitate widespread retinopathy, preretinal and papillary neovascularization and optic atrophy. Anterior segment ischaemia may also occur, manifested as conjunctival and ciliary injection, iris atrophy, cataract and ocular hypotony.

Internal carotid artery insufficiency. Carotid artery stenosis or obstruction is usually secondary to arteriosclerotic or atheromatous vascular disease. Trauma, inflammation and congenital abnormalities are less common causes. Obstruction typically occurs at the bifurcation of the common carotid following thrombosis in the internal carotid at the site of an 'ulcerated' atheromatous plaque. Collaterals developing between the ipsilateral external carotid and ophthalmic arteries may for a time prevent severe ocular ischaemia but they are often ineffectual. Transient failure of vision or loss of the upper or lower field of vision are common symptoms, and small cholesterol or platelet emboli may be detected in the retinal vessels. Unilateral or unequal (right/left) retinopathy, or the presence of impacted microemboli in the retinal circulation are strong evidence of internal carotid artery disease, and a bruit over the internal carotid artery or reduced central retinal artery pressure on the affected side will confirm the diagnosis. Detailed analysis of the carotid vascular system, including Doppler ultrasound measurement of carotid blood flow, is important in such patients. Severe and prolonged carotid artery insufficiency may cause retinal haemorrhages, microaneurysms, cotton wool spots and neovascularization—a syndrome called stasis retinopathy. A high proportion of patients with carotid stenosis will proceed to hemiplegia if untreated, and surgical removal of localized obstruction may produce a dramatic improvement in cerebral function and resolution of retinopathy.

Ophthalmic artery obstruction

Occlusion of the ophthalmic artery itself is rare and is usually secondary to advanced cranial arteritis (giant cell arteritis, temporal arteritis), arteriosclerosis or atherosclerosis. Less common causes are embolization, polyarteritis, trauma and orbital cellulitis.

Obstruction of the central retinal artery near its origin from the ophthalmic artery produces a picture of central retinal artery occlusion that culminates in dense optic atrophy and severe loss of vision.

Obstruction of the ophthalmic artery proximal to the origin of the posterior ciliary vessels compromises the retinal, choroidal *and* papillary circulations; the clinical features are those of infarction of the optic nerve head (ischaemic optic neuropathy) where the disc is pale, swollen and surrounded by flame-shaped haemorrhages and cotton wool spots. However, only the upper or lower portion of the optic disc may be affected, as seen by fluorescein angiography. Retinal arteries are attenuated and both the retinal and choroidal circulations show marked stasis. Generally there is sudden complete and permanent loss of vision on the affected side. *An immediate ESR should be done to exclude giant cell (temporal) arteritis.* If temporal arteritis is present, an immediate and intensive course of systemic corticosteroids may prevent the occurrence of a similar course of events in the contralateral eye (*see* Chapter 7).

Central retinal artery obstruction

Central retinal artery obstruction is usually due to thrombosis secondary to arteriosclerosis or atheroma, or to an embolus impacted at the level of the lamina cribrosa. Rarer causes include giant cell arteritis, sickle cell disease, polyarteritis nodosa, lupus erythematosus and syphilis. The central retinal artery may be compromised by a high intraocular pressure (e.g. in acute closed-angle glaucoma) or by direct pressure (e.g. transmitted by an anaesthetic mask during general anaesthesia or during repair of a blow-out fracture of the orbit). The patient experiences sudden and severe loss of vision in the affected eye, although this may be preceded by visual obscurations or hemianopic loss of field. If the central retinal artery circulation is quickly re-established, vision may return to normal; however, episodes of amaurosis fugax persisting longer than 20 minutes are unlikely to clear with recovery of vision. Immediately after central retinal artery occlusion, the pupil of the affected eye dilates, the retinal vessels become narrow and the red cell column in arteries and veins may become fragmented, indicating gross vascular stasis. Within a few hours, striate haemorrhages appear and the retina becomes white with the exception of the fovea which remains red (cherry red spot). (A similar cherry red spot may also occur in Tay–Sachs disease, in other gangliosidoses and in certain lipid storage diseases—e.g. Niemann–Pick's disease characterized by accumulation of lipid material in retinal ganglion cells.)

The swelling and oedema resolve over a period of two to three weeks, the ganglion cells disintegrate and optic atrophy ensues. There is some restoration of the retinal circulation although the vessels remain narrowed and eventually show arteriosclerotic changes.

There is no treatment of proven value for established central retinal artery occlusion. Rarely, measures to dislodge the embolus may be successful, including ocular massage, vasodilators and acute ocular decompression by paracentesis. The patient with central retinal artery obstruction should be fully investigated from the point of view of the carotid artery insufficiency, hypertension, diabetes and giant cell arteritis.

Branch retinal artery occlusion

Most branch artery occlusions follow impaction of an embolus at a bifurcation. Such an embolus may disimpact and move to smaller branches, which results in marked recovery of vision particularly if foveal circulation is restored. Branch artery occlusion may also be secondary to advanced arteriosclerosis or follow severe retinal vasculitis (e.g. Behçet's disease or systemic lupus erythematosus). If the macula is involved, the patient becomes aware of sudden loss of vision, and a central or paracentral scotoma may remain after the acute episode has resolved. If the upper or lower main branch of the central retinal artery is occluded, an altitudinal hemianopic field defect typically results.

The area of infarcted retina becomes white and opaque, and the margins of the lesion may have a striking flocculent appearance due to obstruction of orthograde (at the distal margin) or retrograde (at the side nearest to the optic disc) axoplasmic flow. The affected arteries are narrowed, and fine superficial haemorrhages may surround the lesion. Small collaterals may develop but they are usually of little consequence on these end-arteries.

Branch retinal vein obstruction

Branch vein occlusion affects elderly or hypertensive individuals and occurs almost exclusively at arteriovenous junctions where the vessels share a common adventitial coat. The superotemporal fundus is a particularly common location as there are more arteriovenous crossings here than elsewhere (*see* Plate 10.6). Most vein occlusions are incomplete, as shown by fluorescein angiography. However, once flow has decreased to a certain critical level a series of events occurs leading to ischaemia of the involved microvasculature. The vein distal to the point of obstruction is dark, dilated and tortuous; proximally it is attenuated and may be partially collapsed. Widespread superficial and deep retinal haemorrhages and oedema occur within the distribution of the obstructed vein, and occasionally extravasated blood erupts through the internal limiting membrane to reach and sometimes fill the vitreous cavity.

Capillary collaterals form almost immediately after the acute venous occlusion and can be identified on fluorescein angiography. Cotton wool spots, which may be confluent, are common; if the superficial optic disc circulation is implicated, sector oedema of the disc may occur, mimicking papillitis or sectoral ischaemic optic atrophy.

Branch vein occlusions are usually symptomless if the macular circulation is not involved. However, vitreous haemorrhage may occur as a late complication of widespread ischaemia, resulting in preretinal or papillary neovascularization. When the macular or perifoveal circulation is involved, prolonged accumulation of fluid may result in microcystoid degenerative changes with destruction of retinal receptors and loss of vision.

With time, most haemorrhages slowly absorb and cotton wool spots fade. Microaneurysms persist for many years, and incompetent venous *macroaneurysms*, which are a feature of vein occlusion, typically become surrounded by circles of fatty exudates. Affected veins remain dilated and tortuous, and fellow arteries typically show advanced arteriosclerotic changes.

First-order vein occlusions (i.e. occlusions of veins draining half the retina) are often incomplete, and partially relieved by venovenous anastomoses which form across the horizontal meridian. They have a relatively good visual prognosis although there may be associated glaucoma.

The treatment of vein occlusion is largely devoted to the management of complications. Vitreous haemorrhage secondary to preretinal and papillary neovascularization can be contained by laser photocoagulation whereby ischaemic retina is 'killed'. Retinal holes or tears may also be sealed by laser photocoagulation or by appropriate retinal detachment surgery. Extramacular areas of chronic intraretinal oedema can also be easily ablated by laser photocoagulation with preservation of visual functions.

Central retinal vein obstruction

Central retinal vein obstruction occurs at the level of the lamina cribrosa where the central retinal artery and vein are juxtaposed in an unyielding adventitial coat (*see* Plate 10.7). Thickening of the vascular media secondary to arteriosclerosis or hypertension probably allows secondary phenomena such as endothelial proliferation and platelet accumulation to precipitate stasis and thrombosis. Central retinal vein occlusion may also be caused by inflammation (e.g. Behçet's disease) and where alterations in blood constituents and viscosity occur (as in polycythaemia, leukaemia) or by external pressure (as in glaucoma).

A relatively benign form of central retinal vein obstruction may occur in younger individuals who may be symptomless or aware of only slight visual change. The veins are dilated, tortuous and dark in colour; however, haemorrhages are relatively few and macular oedema, if present, is typically mild. Fluorescein angiography demonstrates venous stasis and vascular incompetence but the retinal capillary bed is for the most part well perfused. There is good resolution of haemorrhage and oedema, and the visual prognosis for these patients is in general relatively good.

Severe retinal vein obstruction predominantly affects elderly or hypertensive patients usually over the age of 60. There is widespread intraretinal haemorrhage and the veins are dilated, tortuous and dark; cotton wool spots are prominent. There is a general breakdown of the blood–retina barrier and widespread areas of ischaemic retina are present. The prognosis for vision is poor on account of chronic macular oedema and ischaemia of the perifoveal circulation. Rubeosis iridis, secondary glaucoma and phthisis bulbi may also complicate long-standing central retinal vein obstruction.

Anticoagulants, fibrinolytic agents and corticosteroids have all been used in patients with central retinal vein obstruction but their effects are variable and none has been shown to significantly improve the natural course of the disease process. Panretinal photocoagulation may be helpful in preventing or containing the degree and extent of rubeosis iridis and secondary glaucoma.

Systemic hypertension and retinal circulation

The effects of elevated blood pressure are borne principally by small arteries and arterioles which are largely responsible for the peripheral resistance of the circulation. Most retinal vessels are of small order (i.e. 300 μm or less in diameter) and permit the ophthalmologist and physician to analyse the *in vivo* effects of high blood pressure on susceptible vessels. Fluorescein angiography allows an accurate estimate of vessel calibre, provides a sensitive measure of vascular competence and aids evaluation of changes in retinal haemodynamics.

Pathophysiology

The effect of raised intraluminar pressure on walls of the retinal vessels is related to the height of the pressure, its rate of onset and duration, and the condition of the vessel wall prior to the onset of the disease process (e.g. involutionary sclerosis). Normal arterioles respond to a high intraluminar pressure by an initial constriction (up to 50% of their diameter) which is followed by reactive hypertrophy of smooth muscle cells. If hypertension is prolonged, the hypertrophied walls of the vessels undergo a diffuse process of hyalinization, fibrosis and arteriosclerosis. Eventually a balance is established between the intraluminar pressure and the resistance of the vessel wall. When changes have become established they are irreversible.

When blood pressure is raised and maintained at a persistently high level, focal necroses of the arterial wall occur and plasma seeps into the vessel wall through defective endothelial cells (insudation). Occlusion of some arterioles commonly follows, with the development of a cotton wool spot and collapse and closure of the capillary network downstream to the occlusion. This is quickly followed by alterations in the adjacent microvasculature (e.g. microaneurysms and arteriovenous shunts). With time, the cotton wool spots absorb and some reorganization of the collapsed microvasculature takes place.

When blood pressure is markedly elevated for a long time, the retinal microvasculature becomes seriously damaged by ischaemia: widespread haemorrhage, oedema and fatty exudation occur. The retinal vessels show advanced alterations (e.g. fibrinoid degeneration and thrombosis). The optic disc vasculature may also suffer ischaemic changes and become swollen due to the accumulation of axoplasm and oedema from incompetent capillaries in the disc. Such disc swelling may be associated with hypertensive encephalopathy.

Ageing vessels—arteriosclerosis

With increasing age, there is a gradual replacement of smooth muscle cells of the vessel wall by collagen. The arteries become narrow, straight and more rigid. A more exaggerated type of this response is known as arteriosclerosis.

If the intraluminar pressure is elevated in such circumstances, irregular narrowing of the vessel wall takes place at points where smooth muscle cells persist. When the intraluminar pressure is persistently high, closure of some reactive precapillary arterioles occurs, with development of cotton wool spots, retinal oedema and fatty exudates.

Clinical signs (*see* Plates 10.1 to 10.5)

Arterial and arteriolar

Narrowing of the retinal vessels occurs diffusely in young individuals with severe hypertension (accelerated hypertension), acute glomerulonephritis and acute toxaemia of pregnancy. As the vessel wall thickens, the light reflex from the central wall broadens and imparts to the vessel a pale copper colour.

Focal arteriolar constriction and irregular alterations in calibre are the most reliable signs of hypertension. Changes at arteriovenous crossings are especially significant in young individuals. Important findings are constriction, tapering and deflection of the vein at the arteriovenous junction, or the development of an apparent gap between the artery and vein at the crossing. Mild arteriovenous changes in the elderly are less informative as they may merely represent involutionary sclerosis.

Normalization of blood pressure by treatment may have a discernible effect on the retinal arteries or arterioles of young individuals with hypertension of short duration. However, in most cases it is difficult to detect any significant change.

Cotton wool spots (*see* Plates 10.2, 10.3 and 10.5)

Cotton wool spots follow occlusion of a precapillary arteriole. They are white and fluffy and measure about one-third to one-half of a disc diameter in size, predominantly affecting the posterior fundus. They appear within 2–3 days of the acute ischaemic episode and are typically surrounded by microaneurysms and microvascular abnormalities. They fade within a few days and disappear within a few weeks, and generally have little effect on visual functions. The appearance of cotton wool spots in a patient with hypertension is clear evidence that the disease process is not controlled.

Linear or flame-shaped haemorrhages are common in hypertension and usually resolve without complication. The reappearance of fresh haemorrhages is a futher indication that blood pressure has not been normalized.

Retinal oedema and fatty exudates

These represent an outpouring of fluid into the retina which principally accumulates within the outer molecular layer, but often extends to involve all retinal layers. The usual cause is accelerated hypertension. In toxaemia of pregnancy the outpouring of fluid may be so acute as to detach the retina inferiorly, usually in both eyes. Discrete fatty exudates form in the outer molecular layer and often become obvious as the blood pressure is brought under control. Hard exudates in the outer plexiform layer are often arranged in a star-shaped fashion centred on the macula: that is typical of resolving accelerated hypertension.

Optic disc oedema

In severe accelerated hypertension, this usually indicates the presence of advanced involvement of the kidneys, and a poor prognosis for life. The disc oedema is usually mild, and after normalization of blood pressure the oedema resolves although the disc margins may remain blurred. If disc oedema is severe and prolonged, secondary optic atrophy may occur with severe loss of vision. Disc swelling probably represents a combination of ischaemic papillopathy and stasis of orthograde and retrograde axoplasmic flow in the optic nerve fibres.

Choroidal vessel obstruction

Choroidal vessel obstruction may occur in accelerated hypertension and becomes clinically obvious as discrete pigment epithelial defects about one-quarter to one-third of the diameter of the optic disc (Elschnig's spots).

Management

Management of patients found to be hypertensive after evaluation of their fundi requires referral to a physician for investigation and treatment. Life expectancy can be improved by modern treatment of cases with accelerated hypertension even with disc oedema and retinopathy.

Diabetic retinopathy (*see* Plates 10.9 to 10.11)

The number of known diabetics in the population is increasing due to earlier diagnosis and more effective treatment of life-threatening complications. The incidence of known diabetic retinopathy has increased correspondingly and is now one of the major causes of visual handicap and blindness in the developed countries of the world. In England and Wales diabetic retinopathy is responsible for 7% of all new blind registrations.

Background diabetic retinopathy

Very early in the disease, fluorescein angiography can reveal abnormalities of vascular permeability ('leakage') in apparently normal retina. Microaneurysms are one of the first ophthalmoscopically identifiable features of diabetic retinopathy. They appear as small round red or dark blue dots scattered about the posterior fundus, but they may also take the form of saccular or fusiform capillary dilatations and are particularly evident on the venous side of the circulation. Again, fluorescein angiography can demonstrate much greater numbers than are visible with only the ophthalmoscope. There is a slow turnover in the number of microaneurysms, some disappearing while others become hyalinized or thrombosed. Histological studies demonstrate that microaneurysms are outpouchings on the side of the capillary wall lined by attenuated or proliferating cells. There also appears to be a selective loss of pericytes in diabetic capillaries with microaneurysms. Microaneurysms are often surrounded by intraretinal oedema and haloes of fatty exudates. Persistent macular oedema often leads to microcystoid retinal degenerative changes.

Nerve fibre (flame-shaped) and small round haemorrhages are common and as a rule have no serious implications for visual functions as long as the foveal region is not involved. Blotchy haemorrhages may take many months to absorb.

The retinal arteries and arterioles are often narrowed, sheathed or occluded and typically demonstrate arteriosclerotic changes, particularly where they traverse areas of ischaemic retina.

Cotton wool spots are common in diabetic retinopathy and need not necessarily be associated with hypertension although their pathogenesis, histopathology and natural course are similar.

In early diabetic retinopathy there may be generalized dilatation of retinal veins, sometimes very marked. In established disease, typical venous alterations are tortuosity, localized narrowing, beading and loop formation, and reduplication. Branch and central retinal vein occlusions are also common in diabetics.

If there is a markedly elevated plasma triglyceride level, the retinal vessels may have a milky-white appearance, termed 'lipaemia retinalis'. The condition returns rapidly to normal following control of the diabetes.

Proliferative diabetic retinopathy

Proliferative diabetic retinopathy appears in a small proportion of patients. In response to widespread ischaemia, the inner retina and optic disc develop new retinal and papillary vessels. This condition particularly affects young diabetics, and occurs in about one-third of childhood or adolescent diabetics who survive to middle age. Preretinal new vessels are first recognized as abnormal vascular loops or fine capillary-like twigs that arise in the neighbourhood of ischaemic retina. They mostly originate from retinal veins or venules and breach the internal limiting membrane in the vicinity of a major retinal vein. These vessels freely ramify in the preretinal space and gain attachment to both the internal limiting membrane of the retina and the posterior vitreous face. New vessels, unlike normal retinal vessels, are incompetent and leak a protein-rich fluid into the vitreous body, causing liquefaction of the vitreous gel (syneresis) and posterior detachment of the vitreous face. As the posterior vitreous face moves forwards, the unsupported preretinal new vessels may rupture, bleed and impair visual functions.

Papillary neovascularization is similar in most respects to preretinal neovascularization, but forward growth into the vitreous cavity is easier. Developing preretinal and papillary new vessels become associated with a fibrous tissue scaffolding which remains after the new vessels recede or become atrophic. Complications of neovascularization include vitreous haemorrhage, traction effects of fibrous tissue (e.g. retinal holes and detachment), corrugations of the inner retina and preretinal membrane formation.

Occasionally cholesterol crystals are found within the vitreous body (synchysis scintillans) and have a characteristic shimmering appearance. Calcium soaps (asteroid hyalitis) may also be precipitated within the vitreous body, and are apparent as discrete white refractile bodies that move freely within the vitreous cavity on movement of the eyes. Neither of these conditions affects visual function significantly, and they may be present in otherwise healthy eyes or may be associated with conditions other than diabetes.

Ischaemic optic neuropathy may also occur in diabetes following closure of the small papillary vessels. The disc is pale with splinter haemorrhages about its margin, and visual acuity is markedly diminished. Open-angle glaucoma is also more common in diabetics than in the general population, and secondary glaucoma is a common complication of advanced retinal neovascularization and rubeosis iridis, because new vessels and fibrous tissue obstruct the trabecular meshwork (*see* Chapter 5).

Epidemiology

The prevalence of diabetes in the general population is 1–2%. The disease is usually present for about 10 years before retinopathy appears. About

10% of diabetics have significant background retinopathy although with prolonged follow-up and meticulous evaluation (e.g. by fluorescein angiography) up to 70% of diabetics can be shown eventually to develop some vascular changes. Between 1 and 2% of diabetics develop proliferative retinopathy and these patients are more likely to have serious renal and generalized vascular disease. It is estimated that 50% of such patients progress to blindness in five years.

Treatment

Careful diabetic control, particularly in the early years of the disease process, probably influences favourably the development and natural course of retinopathy. Clinical and experimental evidence supports that statement. Therefore, it seems logical to strive for optimum diabetic control in order to minimize the effects of the metabolic abnormality. The introduction of subcutaneous insulin infusions, multiple injections of insulin with improved monitoring, and development of purified insulins are all positive measures in this direction. There is also a relationship between systemic hypertension and the severity of diabetic retinopathy, and optimum control of blood pressure in such patients is clearly advisable.

Xenon arc and laser photocoagulation are effective in patients with papillary neovascularization in whom there is a 60% chance of stabilization of the retinopathy and maintenance of visual functions. Meticulous ablation of leaking retinal vessels may also limit the degree of maculopathy. Hypophysectomy may be helpful in the treatment of an uncommon but florid type of proliferative retinopathy which afflicts some young individuals. This type of retinopathy is often unresponsive to treatment by photocoagulation, but there is a significant morbidity and mortality from pituitary ablation.

The removal of abnormal vitreous (vitrectomy) and peeling of organized preretinal membranes from the retina are now possible, and serve to clear opaque ocular media and relieve traction on the retina. This is particularly important if there is incipient or actual detachment of the macular region.

Developmental abnormalities of the retinal vasculature

Branching and distribution anomalies of the retinal vessels are common, as indeed are precapillary arterial loops where complete or incomplete loops project into the vitreous. Cilioretinal vessels occur in 25–50% of all patients and 5% of such instances are bilateral. Congenital tortuosity is common, with arteries generally affected more than veins. Acquired tortuosity occurs in diabetes, congenital heart disease and venous obstruction, and is occasionally associated with a haemangioma.

Arteriovenous communications

Congenital arteriovenous communications are rare and in most instances represent incidental findings. Small communications are typically stationary and not associated with retinopathy. Larger arteriovenous communications may affect the neighbouring microvasculature because of rapid blood flow, and in rare instances may be associated with intracranial vascular malformations (Wyburn-Mason syndrome).

Retinal vascular abnormalities of unknown cause

Leber's miliary aneurysms affect young individuals, are typically unilateral and may involve any part of the retina. The affected capillary network shows multiple microaneurysms, irregular dilatations and areas of capillary closure. Major retinal arteries and veins also show a variety of alterations, including saccular dilatation and macroaneurysms. Macular degeneration may follow accumulation of fluid and exudates in this region, either from local vascular abnormalities or from more peripherally placed telangiectatic lesions. Laser photocoagulation is helpful in some instances to contain the retinopathy and prevent macular oedema.

In *Coats' disease* the vascular abnormalities are similar but more extensive and associated with widespread accumulation of fluid that may extend within and beneath the retina. Affected blood vessels show a wide variety of abnormalities, including microaneurysms, macroaneurysms, irregularly dilated capillaries and bizarre shunt-like vessels. Macular oedema leading to microcystoid degeneration changes and receptor death is common, and if the telangiectasia is widespread there may be intractable retinal detachment, cataract formation, secondary glaucoma and phthisis bulbi.

Laser photocoagulation may be useful in limited types of the vascular abnormality to reduce the extent of subretinal fluid and exudation.

The differential diagnosis includes infestation of the retina by the larva of the *Toxocara canis* or *cati* which may simulate Coats' disease, especially when a localized retinal detachment is present (*see* Plate 10.12). The worm resides in the intestines of dogs and cats, especially kittens and puppies. Ova in their faeces or vomit contaminate the earth of parks, playgrounds and gardens, so the ova can be ingested and develop into larvae in the child's stomach, then burrow through the stomach wall to reach the circulation and thence the retina (or brain, where they may be a cause of epilepsy).

Advanced Coats' disease may be confused with conditions producing a white fundus reflex ('pseudoglioma')—for example, retinoblastoma, endophthalmitis, Norrie's disease or persistent hyperplastic primary vitreous.

Retinal angiomatosis (von Hippel's disease)

Retinal haemangiomata may be isolated or multiple. They are often small and discrete and found only on screening of the ocular fundus. More commonly they are large, incompetent and associated with haemorrhage or fluid extension into the nearby retina. Most haemangiomata enlarge with time and develop large tortuous feeding and draining vessels. Small haemangiomata should be energetically treated by laser photocoagulation, as the long-term prognosis for such lesions is poor. Larger lesions may be treated by repeated photocoagulation or cryotherapy. Untreated major lesions typically lead to an exudative detachment of the retina and secondary glaucoma.

Retinal haemangiomata may be associated with cerebral and especially cerebellar haemangiomata (von Hippel–Lindau disease). This condition is dominantly inherited and may be associated with haemangiomata of the kidney, pancreas, epididymis and elsewhere. Cerebral haemangiomata require careful evaluation and treatment.

Blood dyscrasias

Blood dyscrasias are associated with changes in the quality and quantity of various blood constituents, which may have a profound effect on the structure and competence of the retinal vasculature. The important physical and chemical changes in the blood responsible for decompensation of the retinal vasculature are the following:

1 Reduction in the oxygen carrying capacity of the blood. For example, anaemia may damage retinal endothelial cells and cause failure of the blood–retina barrier.
2 Increased viscosity of the blood stream. This may lead to stasis and hypoxia (e.g. dysproteinaemia).
3 Alterations in the physical characteristics of the red blood cells. They become more rigid and so are liable to injure the endothelial lining of the vessel walls.
4 Disturbance of normal clotting mechanisms. A wide variety of retinal haemorrhages may result.

Diseases of the red blood cells

Severe anaemia, whether macrocytic, normocytic, aplastic or haemolytic may cause superficial nerve fibre haemorrhages and deeper intraretinal haemorrhages. They are typically circular, with white centres. Segmental retinal oedema may also occur, imparting a hazy character to the retina. Acute blood loss, such as that following a large gastrointestinal haemorrhage, may precipitate optic atrophy and cause severe loss of vision.

Polycythaemia, whether primary or secondary, causes marked dilatation and tortuosity of the retinal blood vessels. When it is severe, scattered superficial and deep haemorrhages occur alongside the engorged veins. In advanced disease, microaneurysms, disc oedema and preretinal and papillary new vessels may occur.

In sickle cell disease, abnormal red blood cells become deformed and rigid when oxygen tension is lowered. The rigid cells injure retinal endothelial cells and become impacted in small channels. The systemic manifestations are most severe in SS sickle cell disease, although the ocular abnormalities may be mild. In SC sickle cell disease, the systemic condition generally runs a milder course but severe proliferative retinopathy may affect the eye.

The peripheral retinal arterioles are narrowed and the corresponding veins are dilated. The intervening capillary network is irregular and may show microaneurysms and widespread areas of ischaemia. Arteriovenous communications develop at the watershed between perfused and non-perfused retina. New vessels arise from the region of arteriovenous communications and proliferate towards the ischaemic retina. The new vessels are often described as fan-shaped and have well-defined feeding arterioles and draining venules. Eventually, the new vessels become enveloped in a mantle of fibrous tissue and lead to complications such as vitreous haemorrhage with later formation of fibrous bands, retinal holes and retinal detachment. Some patients show regression of neovascular fronds over a period of time, and it has been suggested that the atrophic process is the result of 'spontaneous' closure of feeding arterioles (autoinfarction). Small strikingly pigmented chorioretinal scars (black 'sunburst spots') are a common finding and probably result from focal occlusion of choriocapillaris units. Angioid streaks, macular degeneration and glaucoma are uncommon complications of sickle cell disease.

Treatment
Small preretinal neovascular membranes can be directly photocoagulated as they lie on the retina, and fluorescein angiography is helpful in identifying their extent. Larger proliferations are difficult to control, although photocoagulation of feeding arterioles or panphotocoagulation of the retina may be successful. Less accessible foci of neovascularization may be treated by cryotherapy or diathermy. Choroidal neovascularization may complicate intense photocoagulation. Secondary detachment should be treated using standard procedures with particular care to prevent anterior segment ischaemia. There may also be a place for vitrectomy in patients with long-standing vitreous haemorrhage.

Diseases of white blood cells—leukaemia

Retinal vascular alterations are due to the effects of anaemia, increased viscosity and stasis, thrombocytopenia and infiltration of retinal tissues by abnormal white cells. About 9% of children with acute leukaemia suffer some form of eye disease such as retinal haemorrhage or leukaemic infiltration of the optic nerve, retina, iris or orbit.

In severe leukaemia, retinal vessels become dilated and tortuous. Superficial haemorrhages with white centres may appear. Cotton wool spots and greyish patches may develop within the fundus, due to the accumulation of immature and invasive leucocytic cells in the deeper retinal layers. Optic disc oedema may reflect either raised intracranial pressure or direct infiltration of the optic nerve by leukaemic cells.

Diseases of platelets—thrombocytopenia

In both primary and secondary thrombocytopenia, circulating platelets become severely reduced and superficial retinal haemorrhages occur throughout the posterior fundus. Eventually, oedema, fatty exudates and cotton wool spots may occur.

Blood protein disorders—dysproteinaemia and paraproteinaemias

High blood viscosities provoke retinal venous congestion, superficial and deep retinal haemorrhages and multiple microaneurysms. Cotton wool spots, neovascularization and venous occlusion may complicate advanced disease.

Disorders of blood coagulation

Retinal haemorrhages have occasionally been noted in patients with haemophilia or Christmas disease.

11 Trauma

C I Phillips

Prevention

There must be few areas of medicine where successful prevention would be more rewarding in every conceivable way than in trauma. It is one of the commonest causes of serious morbidity and death, especially in the young and active, so it must account for a vast amount of person-years of incapacity. Its sociopsycho-epidemiology is an important problem. Injuries to the eyeball itself often have very serious long-term effects.

General

The injured patient presents some challenging diagnostic problems. As always, every attempt should be made to obtain a satisfactory history. The general casualty officer, as well as the ophthalmic one, who is seeing a patient with swollen eyelids should specifically consider both a blow-out fracture of the floor of the orbit and a fracture of the malar bone, either of which may require urgent operation. Careful palpation along the orbital margin and malar bones to identify any point of marked tenderness or crepitus is more important than an x-ray. Even more important, the eyeball itself should be inspected— gently— to exclude a perforating injury in all patients whose eyelids are closed by oedema. An ophthalmologist's help may be required to part the eyelids with Desmarres retractors under topical anaesthesia.

All doctors and nurses—especially anaesthetists, neurosurgeons, neurologists, physicians, casualty officers, accident and emergency physicians and surgeons—must be aware of the dangers to the cornea if the lids are open or even not quite shut, especially in the unconscious patient: corneal dehydration within an hour or so, ulceration and infection within a day, then panophthalmitis within 2–3 days can quickly evolve in such an eye or, even more tragically, eyes. The simple application of a piece of adhesive tape to hold the upper lid shut down to the lower is all that is required to prevent a disaster. Alternatively, an antibiotic ointment three to four times daily (in large amounts at night) may suffice.

Likewise the ophthalmologist receiving a patient in his accident and emergency department or his wards with an injury to the eye or orbit should look at his patient generally to exclude other injuries—from a fractured ankle or ribs, ruptured liver or spleen to a fractured skull with brain injury.

One particularly subtle injury may occur, especially in children who often cannot or will not give a history. An innocent-seeming small wound of the upper lid may in fact be an entry wound of a thin stick on which the child has fallen; and the stick may have entered the orbit *and* eyeball, or may have pierced the thin roof of the orbit to enter the frontal lobes of the brain. And a piece of the stick may have been left behind. Lift the upper lid to inspect as much as possible of the eyeball, and test the visual acuity: watch for signs of intracranial injury even if an x-ray shows no fracture or foreign body.

Antibiotics are often required as part of the treatment. Tetanus antiserum may be indicated if contamination is likely—it must later be followed by a course of active immunization; a booster of tetanus toxoid is often appropriate in those already actively immunized.

Unilateral/Bilateral

One very fortunate property of injuries is that they are usually unilateral; provided that the other eye does not have strabismic amblyopia or some other disease, the patient's situation is not disastrous, and he seldom, if ever, needs to change his occupation. Because of this, some surgeons prefer to avoid corneal grafts and/or cataract extractions in unilateral cases although many rate binocular vision more highly. On the other hand, severe injuries of the eye have a poor prognosis and so in a bilateral case (e.g. a windscreen injury in a motor accident) the result can be tragic blindness.

Eyelids

Lacerated wounds are common and are usually simple to suture. If the lower lacrimal canaliculus is torn, its repair is difficult, and permanent epiphora may result. Damage to the upper canaliculus is unimportant. Distortion of the eyelashes (trichiasis) is a complication which must be prevented if at all possible. If these rub on the cornea or conjunctiva, they should be epilated or permanently eliminated by electrolysis.

Conjunctival foreign bodies

These must be one of the commonest of all injuries, with a typical history of a sudden onset of pain in the eye, when the patient is walking past a building site in a wind. Usually the foreign body gravitates into the lower fornix where it can be easily seen with a good light (a focusing torch is useful) and removed with a sterile cotton wool swab or at least a clean handkerchief.

Subtarsal foreign bodies

The pain in this case is partly due to sensitivity of the conjunctiva—for example, on the undersurface of the upper lid where the foreign body usually is found in the sulcus a few millimetres behind, and parallel to, the lid margin (*see* Fig 11.1 for technique of removal). The pain is also worse on blinking because of the rubbing of the foreign body over the surface of the very sensitive cornea. Areas of corneal epithelial damage can be shown up by fluorescein eyedrops. After removal, framycetin ointment (Soframycin) twice daily for 2–3 days will act as a lubricant and also help to prevent infection.

Corneal foreign bodies

These often have the same history as conjunctival and subtarsal foreign bodies, but may be occupational—particles from a buff or any other producer of small blunt particles at high speed. (*Do not miss intraocular foreign bodies:* see *below*.) The particles may be quite small and white, so a close-up search of the whole cornea (NB lift the upper lid) with a bright focused light is often necessary; otherwise this simple diagnosis is easy to miss. Removal is usually easy, after instillation of amethocaine or other topical anaesthetic eyedrops, with a sterile cotton wool swab on a stick. If the foreign body is immovable, a sterile disposable needle on a disposable syringe as a handle is useful—but if this is required, specialist treatment may be advisable. Again, framycetin ointment (Soframycin) or similar should be given twice daily, and a pad taped over the eye to keep the

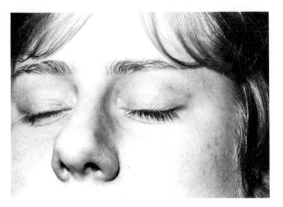

Fig 11.1 Technique of eversion of left upper lid and removal of subtarsal foreign body.

(a) The patient lies on a couch with one thin pillow. The operator washes his hands thoroughly and scrubs his nails, then stands behind the top of the patient's head. The patient is asked to look down towards her feet.

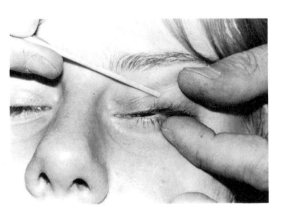

(b) The free end of a sterile swabstick in the operator's right hand is placed 5–6 mm above the lash margin (i.e. at the upper border of the tarsal plate) to act as a fulcrum round which the left thumb and finger rotate the upper lid. The operator's left thumb pulls the skin of the upper lid laterally and slightly upwards to disengage the lid margin from the eyeball.

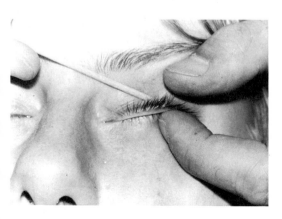

(c) The left forefinger is used to push the margin of the lower lid up underneath the edge of the upper lid. Moderate pressure by the left thumb contributes to the fulcrum being applied by the swabstick, both of which push the upper margin of the upper lid's tarsal plate downwards until

(d) The upper lid turns inside out.

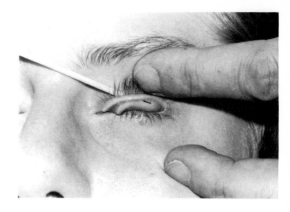

(e) The other end of the swabstick (sterile) is then used to remove any subtarsal foreign body.

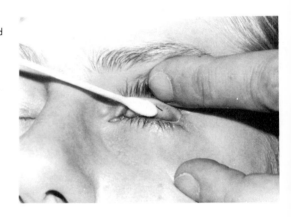

(f) Finally the margin of the lower lid is used as a fixed point on to which the edge of the everted tarsal plate is pressed so that the upper lid flips back into its normal position.

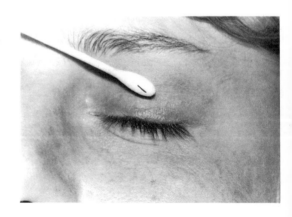

upper lid shut for two to three days. About two days after the foreign body has been removed, the eye should be inspected again to ensure that an infected corneal ulcer is not developing.

Corneal ulcer

Infection is a rare but serious complication after trivial injury of the cornea and is usually due to pyogenic organisms (e.g. staphylococci). The infection should *never* be introduced by the doctor's manipulations, instruments or eyedrops. He should scrub thoroughly before touching or treating the patient's eye, his instruments must be sterile and he should use single-dose containers for eyedrops (or a fresh bottle or tube of ointment) if the patient is to take it with him (e.g. Soframycin Eye Ointment). Other organisms found in corneal ulcers are viruses and, especially in agricultural injuries, fungi.

The edges and bed of an early corneal ulcer are whitish-grey and there is marked conjunctival hyperaemia, particularly at the nearby part of the limbus—or all round the limbus if the ulcer is central (*see* Plate 11.1a). The slough is the result of migration of leucocytes through the corneal stroma from the limbus in response to inflammatory 'toxins'. These toxins also diffuse into the anterior chamber and stimulate an exudation of white cells etc. from the iris; this inflammatory exudate gravitates to the bottom of the anterior chamber where it accumulates and may be visible as a hypopyon (Greek *hypo*, below; *pyon*, pus) (*see* Plate 11.1b). The organisms may progress into the anterior chamber which fills with pus, then into the vitreous chamber to produce a septic panophthalmitis—which has a poor prognosis for vision. Such an eye may have to be enucleated (completely removed with cutting of the optic nerve) or eviscerated (the contents of the scleral envelope scraped out after removal of the cornea). Early intensive treatment may be successful but at the very least a corneal opacity will result.

Corneal abrasion

This follows a glancing injury with, say, a newspaper or a child's finger. The area deprived of epithelium is usually invisible unless stained with fluorescein eyedrops (*see* Plate 11.2). Framycetin ointment (Soframycin) with a protective pad for a few days helps to expedite Nature's healing process—again, secondary infection is *the* great danger.

Recurrent corneal abrasion

This is an interesting but uncommon complication of apparently trivial injury. After a variable interval (weeks or months) following a corneal abrasion the patient wakes up with pain in the eye identical with the original symptoms but it lasts 15–30 minutes. Frequency varies from two or three times weekly to once in every few months. Presumably the epithelium which has regrown over the original abrasion has not achieved a good enough hold on the underlying Bowman's membrane. On waking, the patient opens his eyes and the unstable area of epithelium (? stuck to the upper lid during the night) is lifted off like a door opening. The presence of a hinge is presumed—it allows the flap of epithelium to fall back into place a few minutes after symptoms have started.

Treatment is conservative; reassurance may be required. Nightly framycetin ointment (Soframycin) is usually sufficient for a few weeks and spontaneous resolution will occur. Troublesome symptoms may require carbolization of the area (which is difficult to identify) to produce more damage so that the healing epithelium will obtain a more firm hold on the underlying cornea.

Chemical burns

Chemical burns of the cornea and conjunctiva are serious, and most cases are avoidable.

Alkalis

Lime burns occur when carelessly handled dry lime on a building site is blown into one eye—or, quite tragically, both eyes. As an emergency measure, tap water should be irrigated over the eyeball with the lids held apart and any solid pieces of lime picked off. The patient should be immediately transferred to hospital where local or general anaesthesia and ophthalmic instruments will allow more detailed toilette, with special attention to the conjunctival fornices. Serious complications often ensue. The two surfaces of conjunctiva (on the lids and on the eyeball, fully into the depths of the fornices) are denuded of epithelium and become cicatrized together, making the eyelids stick to the eyeballs (symblepharon) sometimes in a 'half open' position, thus exposing the cornea. Treating this surgically, with grafts of mucous membrane from the mouth, is very difficult.

The cornea suffers even more than would be expected. Obviously, cicatrization and opacification will result. Along with these, vascularization is also very typical of lime burns. The new blood vessels are accompanied by lymphatics, both of which make the prognosis for corneal grafting very poor, because of the increased risk of host–graft reaction.

A chronic, progressively deeper corneal ulcer often develops after lime burns. The mechanism is the removal of inhibition of collagenase which progressively digests corneal collagen. Cystein eyedrops may halt the process.

Acid

Acid burns produce similar results to alkalis but without the *progressive* ulceration.

Eyeball concussion

Concussion of the eyeball is also a very common injury, especially in children—balls being the main cause, and not entirely preventable! Most cases are minor, and recovery is complete.

A more severe concussion may cause a hyphaema—i.e. an extravasation of blood from around the base of the iris which, like hypopyon, gravitates to the bottom of the anterior chamber and shows a horizontal fluid level on top. (Hyphaema is from the Greek: *hypo*, below; *haema*, blood.) It may be only just visible or it may fill the anterior chamber. Raised intraocular pressure may occur either because the trabecular meshwork is concussed and quite possibly swollen, or because the hyphaema silts up the drainage channels in the trabecular meshwork. Most hyphaemas absorb in a few days but the patient should be almost confined to bed for 5–7 days lest a secondary, much bigger hyphaema occur, presumably because blood clots in the damaged vessels are digested away at that interval. The secondary hyphaema is usually much larger and has a much more serious prognosis; surgical evacuation is usually necessary to prevent intractable glaucoma.

Cataract sooner or later may follow a severe concussion of the eyeball with or without partial or complete dislocation of the lens. Macular oedema with reduced visual acuity for a few days is common. A contre-coup mechanism as in head injuries probably accounts for ruptures in the choroid at the posterior pole, typically concentric with the disc. Rupture of the overlying retina also often occurs, sometimes with disastrous results on visual acuity but with retained normal peripheral fields.

Perforating injury

Perforating injuries by sharp objects (e.g. knives) tend to affect the anterior segment of the eyeball and are serious. An iris prolapse frequently occurs. Even the most minor puncture wound of the capsule of the lens will produce progressive cataract (opacification of the lens) within a few days. The anterior eyeball behind the lens is also sometimes involved, with escape of vitreous—a clear semi-fluid substance like white of egg.

Treatment is excision of any iris prolapse, generous removal of escaping vitreous or anterior vitrectomy with a suction-cutter and fluid infusion, and careful suturing of the corneoscleral wounds under the operation microscope. Antibiotics systemically and topically will reduce the risk of sepsis. The damaged lens may be removed at the same time or a few weeks or months later. Corneal scarring and fibrous bands in the pupil area and also in the vitreous cavity are a common end-result: the bands may be excised–aspirated by a suction-cutting (plus infusion) cannula—a vitrectomy—while the corneal irregularity may be susceptible to a contact lens (to treat also the aphakia) or a corneal graft. However, some surgeons prefer a more conservative attitude if the fellow eye is normal.

Sympathetic ophthalmitis

This is one of the most fascinating diseases in the whole of medicine. After a perforating injury of one eye, very occasionally *both eyes* develop an inflammation of the *whole uveal tract* (i.e. iris, ciliary body and choroid). It has never been known to occur if the 'exciting' (i.e. injured) eye is removed within nine days of the perforating injury. The peak incidence is three months after the injury, though it is said that the risk never diminishes to zero. Accordingly, ophthalmologists have to decide by the eighth or ninth day whether a badly injured eye with a very poor ultimate prognosis for vision is better removed rather than to take the small risk of the tragedy of this diabolical disease. Treatment with anti-inflammatory drugs, especially cortisone, may slow down the progression to ultimate blindness—which may take some years or even a decade or so to evolve. The exciting eye is generally removed as soon as the disease is suspected to be developing but the operation is usually of no avail. The commonest perforating injury of the eyeball, of course, is an intraocular operation (e.g. for cataract or glaucoma) and so an occasional case (around 1 in 10 000 cases, perhaps) has a tragic ending.

Clinically, there is a low-grade iridocyclitis plus mild choroiditis in both eyes with all their usual complications, especially cataract and glaucoma. Histologically, the disease is characteristic.

The mechanism is probably a lymphocytic (delayed hypersensitivity) reaction of the body's reticuloendothelial system to its own uveal tissue which it regards as 'not self' because the uvea has been incarcerated inside the walls of the lymphatic-less eyeball from a time early in intrauterine life. That hypothesis, however, fails to explain why all cases of perforating injury and intraocular operations do not develop sympathetic ophthalmitis! An individual susceptibility of unknown cause is postulated in these rare cases.

Intraocular foreign body

The diagnosis is sometimes missed and should be suspected from the history—for example, a man using a hammer and chisel or working at a lathe without goggles feels a transient sensation of foreign body in one eye and none can be found in the cornea or conjunctival sac. The visual acuity may be normal if the entry has been through conjunctiva and sclera and so has avoided the lens. A conjunctival–scleral entry wound is often invisible. The visual acuity will be subnormal if the capsule or lens itself has been damaged and a cataract is developing; an entry wound of a small foreign body through the cornea may require a slit-lamp microscope to be seen. A likely history demands an x-ray which will exclude a radio-opaque foreign body. Most are iron-containing and can be fairly easily removed by a magnet, with or without vitrectomy, although the sequelae are like those of any perforating injury. A piece of metal from a lathe is unlikely to produce infection because its heat sterilized it at the start of its journey. A fragment from a hammer or chisel (it is less often from the material being chiselled) is cold and so is more likely to carry a variety of organisms into the eyeball.

Unilateral cataract

This is usually traumatic in origin, due to concussion or penetrating injury of the eyeball, or intraocular foreign body. Although the fellow eye usually has good vision, the patient may feel more or less handicapped by his unilateral cataract which causes him loss of binocularity and loss of an area of field on that side. Within a few months his pupil can usually be seen to be white, and after some years his cataract may become 'hypermature'—i.e. swollen (with a risk of closed-angle glaucoma of a sort) or fluid (with a risk of an iridocyclitis due to outward diffusion of degenerated products of the lens). The eye will tend to develop a divergent squint if the patient is adult: a convergent squint will occur if the patient is a child under, say, 7 years. Most ophthalmologists advise a cataract extraction, which will prevent some of these possible complications but will raise others (apart from the small risks of the operation itself).

The strong convex spectacle lens of about 10 dioptres required for the aphakic eye will produce an image 25% larger than on the normal side (if the fellow eye is emmetropic)—which causes intolerable diplopia so the patient will not wear such spectacles. A contact lens, being nearer the nodal point of the eye, reduces the difference in image sizes to around 8%, and, surprisingly, good binocular vision (for distance) can be achieved. However, the patient may derive little benefit from his unilateral contact lens and about half of such patients give up wearing the lens within a few months, and so eventually develop a squint. Theoretically the best solution to the problem is the insertion of an acrylic intraocular lens to replace the cataractous lens, provided that the original injury did not cause significant other damage to the cornea, iris or posterior segment to preclude its use. These intraocular lenses, however, carry their own extra risks, such as damage to corneal endothelium, dislocation or infection.

12 Eyelids

A G Tyers and J R O Collin

Introduction

The eyelids protect the eyes. Spontaneous blinking sweeps away microscopic débris and moistens the eyes with tears. A dust fragment or bright light stimulates reflex blinking, and during sleep the eyes are protected by continuous eyelid closure. Without eyelids, the combined effect of desiccation and repeated minor trauma would soon lead to painful blindness. Neglected lid disease may have the same disastrous result.

To function efficiently, the lids must be smooth and, where they are in contact with the eye, they must close completely and there must be an adequate flow of tears. Lid diseases frequently affect one or more of these factors and only *prompt* treatment will prevent complications leading to blindness.

The layers of an eyelid can be conveniently grouped into a posterior lamella (conjunctiva and tarsal plate) and an anterior lamella (orbicularis muscle and skin). The tarsal plate largely determines the shape of the eyelid, and posterior lamellar disease may distort the lid and scar its posterior surface, causing abrasion of the cornea. Tear production may also be compromised. Anterior lamellar disease more commonly interferes with proper lid closure, risking eye exposure.

Other eyelid diseases (e.g. small tumours) may not affect eyelid function but require treatment because of their natural history or cosmetic effect.

Malpositions of the eyelid

Entropion (*see* Plate 12.1)

Definition   Inward turning of the margin of the eyelid.

Classification   Senile
Cicatricial
Congenital

Whatever the aetiology, an entropion allows the lashes to abrade the eye, causing discomfort and eventual corneal scarring.

Senile entropion is common and results from laxity of the lower lid and orbital tissues with ageing. Surgery is often required with the aim of tightening the lax tissues, and many operations for senile entropion have been described. Because the underlying process of involution is progressive, there is a chance of recurrence even after initially successful surgery. Temporary relief while awaiting surgery may be obtained by taping the lower eyelid skin with a downward pull to the cheek to maintain eversion.

Cicatricial entropion is due to contraction of scar tissue in the posterior lamella and may affect upper or lower lid. The commonest causes are chemical burns—strong alkali burns, in particular, lead to extensive scarring—and irradiation. Other diseases causing posterior lamellar scarring include erythema multiforme, cicatrizing conjunctival pemphigoid and infections such as pseudomembranous conjunctivitis and trachoma. Tear flow is often compromised by the scarring, so artificial tears (e.g. hypromellose drops) are frequently needed. Surgery aims to evert the lid margin and lengthen the contracted posterior lamella.

Congenital entropion is rare, and is due to excess skin and muscle close to the margin of the lower lid. Excision of the excess tissues corrects the condition.

Eyelash abnormalities

In entropion, although the lashes abrade the cornea, once the lid is everted the lashes return to their normal position. There are three other conditions, however, in which the lashes themselves are abnormal in direction or site and cause corneal discomfort and scarring.

Trichiasis
Scarring at the lid margin distorts the direction of the lash follicles so that some may grow posteriorly towards the eye.

Metaplastic lashes
Certain diseases (e.g. erythema multiforme) are associated with abnormal lashes which grow from the meibomian orifices and abrade the cornea.

Distichiasis
In this rare congenital lid abnormality, metaplastic lashes grow from most of the meibomian orifices.

Treatment of these conditions is best with cryotherapy. Liquid nitrogen spray is used to achieve a temperature of −20°C which kills the lash follicles. Epidermis is less sensitive to this temperature, and techniques are available for protection of the normal lashes.

Ectropion (Fig 12.1)

Definition	Outward turning of the margin of the eyelid.
Classification	Senile
	Cicatricial
	Paralytic

Whatever the aetiology, an ectropion often prevents proper lid closure, with a risk of exposure of the eye. Tears fail to drain into the everted lacrimal punctum, and patients complain of troublesome watering of the eye (epiphora).

Senile ectropion is due to involutional laxity of the tissues and, as in senile entropion, affects only the lower lid. Surgery aims to tighten the eyelid horizontally by excision of a full-thickness triangular wedge of eyelid with the base on the lid margin.

Cicatricial ectropion is equally common in the lower and upper lids. It is due to contraction of scar tissue in the anterior eyelid lamella. Scars may be linear (e.g. following a laceration) or diffuse (e.g. after a burn). Contraction in linear scars is treated surgically with a Z-plasty. Diffuse scars (Fig 12.2) are corrected with a skin graft after the tension has been relieved. Thermal burns cause rapid contraction of the thin eyelid skin, and a skin graft may be needed within 24 hours of the injury to protect the eye from exposure (Fig 12.3).

Paralytic ectropion is due to paralysis of the orbicularis muscle as part of a facial palsy. The unsupported lower eyelid stretches and everts. The risk of exposure is especially great because the upper lid also is unable to close. Normal eyelid closure is accompanied by upward movement of the eye—Bell's phenomenon. It is not affected in an isolated facial palsy and provides the only remaining protection for the cornea.

Exposure of the eye

Whenever the eyelids are prevented from closing properly, the exposed eye is at risk from desiccation and repeated minor trauma. Advanced

Fig 12.1 Left senile ectropion.

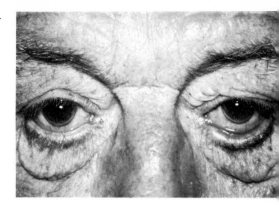

Fig 12.2 Diffuse scar below the lateral part of the right lower lid, causing cicatricial ectropion.

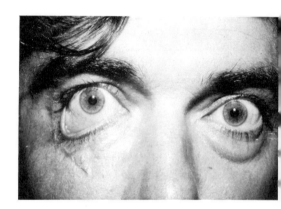

Fig 12.3 Flash burn which has caused contraction of the thin lid skin, resulting in inability to close the eyes. Note that Bell's phenomenon is present.

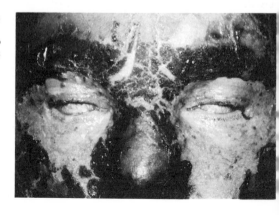

senile ectropion, facial palsy, contracted anterior lamellar scars and extreme proptosis are the commonest causes. The eye is particularly at risk if tear flow is also reduced, or the cornea is anaesthetic due to poor Vth cranial nerve function.

The main aims in management are to keep the eye moist and protected. A normal Bell's phenomenon may achieve this but supplementary drops (e.g. hypromellose) and ointment are usually needed. If exposure is severe, a laboratory watchglass or similar convex shield taped to the skin around the eye effectively retains moisture and provides protection, but surgery to reduce the area of eye exposure between the lids is often required. The lids may be sutured together laterally with a lateral tarsorrhaphy (Fig 12.4) and a contact lens may be used to provide extra protection. (In tarsorrhaphy the surgeon removes the epithelial surface along a section of the upper lid margin *and* a corresponding section of the lower lid margin, and stitches the two raw surfaces together; after a week or so, the two sections become permanently joined by scar tissue.)

In thyroid eye disease proptosis is compounded by lid retraction which may be severe. A lateral tarsorrhaphy usually provides adequate protection of the eye from exposure but a more cosmetic and effective approach is the use of donor sclera or fascia lata to lengthen the posterior lamellae of upper and lower lids.

Ptosis (Fig 12.5)

Definition	Drooping of the upper eyelids.
Classification	Congenital
	Acquired

Ptosis not only causes a cosmetic deformity but also restricts the vision in up-gaze and in the primary position if severe. This is important in children, who tend to adopt an uncomfortable head-back posture to improve vision and occasionally develop amblyopia on the affected side.

Congenital ptosis is uncommon. It is present from birth and is most frequently due to a dystrophy of the levator palpebrae superioris muscle. At least 80% of all cases of ptosis are congenital, the majority are unilateral and about 10% have an associated weakness of the superior rectus muscle. There is no spontaneous improvement and treatment is surgical, usually at about the age of 4 years when the child can be properly assessed, unless obstructed vision makes earlier surgery necessary. Function in the levator muscle determines the choice of operation. A well-functioning muscle is shortened to lift the lid, but if function is poor, autogenous fascia lata is used as a sling between the lid and the frontalis muscle.

Fig 12.4 Left eye. Lateral tarsorrhaphy.

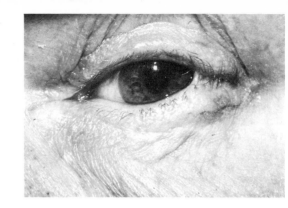

Fig 12.5 Left congenital ptosis.

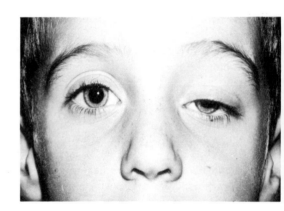

Fig 12.6 Epicanthic folds.

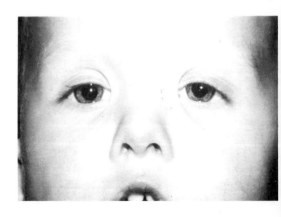

Acquired ptosis may result from *mechanical* causes such as a laceration or senile disinsertion of the levator muscle aponeurosis, *neurogenic* causes as in Horner's syndrome or a IIIrd cranial nerve palsy, or *myogenic* causes such as myasthenia gravis, progressive external ophthalmoplegia and myotonic dystrophy.

Mechanical acquired ptosis is treated surgically in an attempt to restore the normal anatomy of the levator muscle. Other causes frequently leave the levator with poor residual function and so a fascia lata sling may be needed. However, simple external devices, such as modified spectacles or special contact lenses with a shelf to support the lid, are often found to be more satisfactory.

Dermatochalasis

Thin eyelid skin stretches with advancing age, causing 'baggy' eyelids. In addition, orbital fat may herniate through the weak orbital septum into the lids. The operation of blepharoplasty aims to remove excess skin and fat.

Epicanthus

These congenital vertical folds of skin (Fig 12.6; *see also* Fig 3.4) partly cover the medial canthus and tend to improve with facial development. They are normal in Eastern races but when they occur in a Caucasian child the appearance may be mistaken for a convergent squint. Exclusion of a true squint is important so that the parents can be reassured. Surgery is not advised for persistent epicanthic folds, unless severe, until the age of 8–10 years when the effect of facial development, particularly that of the bridge of the nose, can be assessed.

Inflammations

Blepharitis

Definition	Inflammation of the eyelid margin.
Classification	Squamous
	Ulcerative
	Allergic

Squamous blepharitis is usually associated with dandruff and seborrhoeic dermatitis. It causes mild irritation of the lid margin and occurs from adolescence onwards. Fine desquamated flakes are found along the lash roots and there is no ulceration.

Ulcerative blepharitis is due to staphylococcal infection and often begins in childhood. The lid margins are ulcerated and there is low-grade conjunctivitis.

Treatment of squamous and of ulcerative blepharitis is the same. The lid margins are cleaned twice daily with saline to remove crusts and then chloramphenicol (Chloromycetin) ointment is applied close to the lash roots. Treatment continues for 10–14 days.

Allergic blepharitis is caused by chemical irritants such as eyedrops or cosmetics. The inflammation resolves when the cause is removed, and may be hastened with hydrocortisone 1% ointment twice daily for about five days.

Chalazion

Definition   A chronic inflammatory granuloma within a meibomian gland of the tarsal plate caused by retention of the secretion of the gland. Note that this is not a true cyst: the wall consists of granulation tissue with giant cells, rather like tuberculous granulation tissue!

A chalazion begins as a small nodule within the tarsal plate and enlarges slowly, usually without acute inflammation or pain. Chalazions are very common in adults and older children, and the treatment is incision through the conjunctiva with curettage of the contents. Recurrences in other meibomian glands are not uncommon.

Internal hordeolum (syn. acute chalazion)

Definition   An acute infection of a meibomian gland usually due to *Staphylococcus aureus* (*see* Plate 12.2).

The infected tarsal gland presents with acute localized swelling, redness and pain in the eyelid. It may progress towards abscess formation with rupture into the skin or conjunctiva, or gradually resolve leaving a small nodule in the tarsus. Chloramphenicol ointment is prescribed twice daily to control the infection, and local heat is applied to encourage drainage. Incision may be necessary.

External hordeolum (syn. 'stye')

Definition   A suppurative infection of a lash follicle and its sebaceous gland, usually due to *Staphylococcus aureus*.

A stye may be confused with an internal hordeolum but is closer to the lash roots and has no tendency to expand posteriorly into the conjunctival surface of the lid. The acute localized swelling usually progresses and ruptures anteriorly close to the lash roots. Hot compresses are combined with chloramphenicol ointment and removal of the eyelash. An abscess is incised.

Skin infections

Herpes simplex

Herpes simplex virus may affect the skin, conjunctiva or cornea but, unlike herpes zoster virus (*see* below), is not restricted to the distribution of branches of sensory nerves. Primary infection occurs in childhood as crops of vesicles on the skin of the face. The eye is usually not involved although a conjunctivitis is seen occasionally. Recurrent infection occurs throughout life and the cornea may be involved. The typical corneal appearance is of a branching 'dendritic' ulcer which stains with fluorescein. Bilateral corneal involvement is uncommon, surprisingly.

The skin lesions may be treated with an antiviral ointment such as idoxuridine or adenine arabinoside or acyclovir four or five times daily. Steroids are contraindicated in herpes simplex infections.

Herpes zoster

Herpes zoster virus infects the dorsal roots of extramedullary ganglia of cranial nerves and causes pain and a vesicular rash in the distribution of the involved nerve. Infection of the ophthalmic division of the Vth cranial nerve involves the upper eyelid, and the forehead and scalp on the same side (Fig 12.7). Fifty per cent of patients also have small corneal ulcers

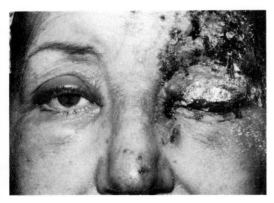

Fig 12.7 Herpes zoster ophthalmicus. Note that the rash extends to the tip of the nose.

and an iritis which is particularly likely if the rash extends to the tip of the nose. Infection in the maxillary division of the Vth cranial nerve involves the lower eyelid but not the eye. Attacks are heralded by pain in the distribution of the infected nerve several days before the rash appears. A few patients suffer prolonged pain—post-herpetic neuralgia.

The skin rash is treated with idoxuridine skin ointment for four days, and then a bland ointment while the crusts separate and the swelling resolves. If the eye is involved, steroid eyedrops (e.g. prednisolone, Predsol) are given four times daily; the pupil should be dilated if an iritis is present although posterior synechiae are uncommon. Post-herpetic neuralgia is best treated with carbamazepine orally.

Tumours

The skin of the eyelids is subject to all tumours found in the skin elsewhere.

Benign tumours (e.g. basal and squamous cell papillomata) appear as slow-growing sessile nodules (Fig 12.8) which almost never become malignant. If they do not involve the lid margin they are easily removed with a minimum of surrounding skin. If the lid margin is involved, careful reconstruction of the lid is required after excision of the tumour to prevent a marginal notch.

Naevi are flat pigmented spots present from childhood. They are seen in the skin and occasionally in the conjunctiva. No treatment is required; although malignant change does occur, this is rare. A pigmented lesion with greater malignant potential is *premalignant melanosis.* This acquired pigmentation appears in middle age, usually in the conjunctiva and often spreads over the lid margin to the skin of the eyelid. It is flat, diffuse and variably pigmented. Only observation is needed unless any part of the lesion darkens in colour and becomes raised, signifying probable

Fig 12.8 Squamous papilloma of lower lid.

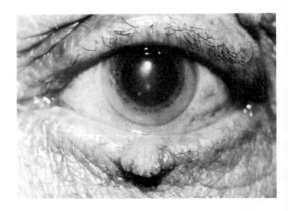

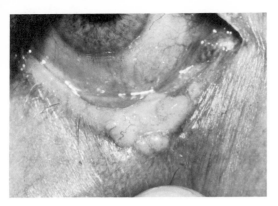

Fig 12.9 Basal cell carcinoma at the lid margin.

malignant change. A congenital form of melanosis is seen in dark-skinned races but it is non-progressive and has little malignant potential.

In addition to the benign tumours, flat waxy deposits are commonly found in the skin of the inner ends of the lids in association with raised blood cholesterol level. These are *xanthelasmata* (*see* Plate 12.3), and the deposits may be removed for cosmetic reasons.

Malignant tumours are relatively common in the eyelids. Basal cell and squamous cell carcinomata are often indistinguishable without biopsy. They appear as sessile nodules (Fig 12.9), often close to the lid margin, which enlarge over a year or so and may ulcerate and bleed. Local excision is curative in 95% and is the treatment of choice if the tumour is on the eyelid. Radiotherapy is of value for small basal cell carcinomata in nearby skin, and ones which have extended into the tissues of the orbit where they are beyond the reach of conservative surgery. Squamous cell carcinomata are not as sensitive to irradiation, and occasionally metastasize to local lymph nodes.

Malignant melanomata are uncommon in the lid but may be seen occasionally, either in the skin or in the conjunctiva. They arise from pre-existing benign naevi, areas of premalignant melanosis and possibly *de novo*. Wide local excision is the treatment of choice although radiotherapy may be used in those arising in premalignant melanosis. Prognosis must be guarded, but is generally better than malignant melanomas of the trunk or limbs.

Examination of the eyelids

1   Is there obvious pathology?

Look at the external lid surface and surrounding facial skin for signs of disease—tumours, scars, inflammation.

2   Is the position of the lid normal?

With the eyes open, look for ptosis, lid retraction, entropion, ectropion, proptosis.

3   Is the movement of the lids normal?

Check that the lids open and close normally.

The levator muscle lifts the upper lid. To assess levator function the action of the frontalis muscle must be eliminated first by firm pressure above the brow with a thumb. If the patient now looks up and down the excursion of the upper lid is due only to levator, and should be 15–18 mm in the normal lid. It is often reduced in ptosis.

The orbicularis oculi muscle closes the lids. Incomplete closure may be due to weakness of the muscle or there may be a mechanical restriction— a notch in the lid margin or a contracted scar.

If the lid closure is incomplete it is important to ensure that the eye is adequately protected. Look for Bell's phenomenon by asking the patient to close the eyes. Inspect the cornea for signs of an abrasion or ulcer.

4   What is the cause of the abnormality?

Anterior lamellar pathology is usually obvious.

The posterior surface of the *lower* lid is easily seen.

To evert the *upper* lid ask the patient to look down, grasp the lashes between thumb and forefinger, and pull downwards. About mid-way between the lashes and the brow (at the upper border of the tarsal plate), depress the lid with a glass rod (or pen), and evert the lid over it. As long as the patient maintains downgaze the lid can be kept everted. Look for scarring, distortion or tumours.

13

The Orbit and Proptosis

A L Crombie

Applied anatomy

The orbits are two bony cavities in the skull. The medial walls are parallel to each other on either side of the nose, and the lateral walls are at an angle of 45 degrees to each other. The volume of an orbit is approximately 35–40 ml and its shape is roughly that of a pyramid on its side, the base being to the front. 'Covering' the base of the pyramid is a fibrous sheet of tissue, the orbital septum, which holds in place the eyeball and the rest of the orbital contents—extraocular muscles, nerves, blood vessels and fat. The maxillary sinuses lie below the orbits, the ethmoid sinuses lie medial to them, while the frontal sinuses and frontal lobes of the brain lie above the orbits. The lacrimal gland lies in the upper outer part of the orbit, and the lacrimal sac at the lower inner part of the orbit. The medial wall and the floor of each orbit are thinner than the other walls and roof, and the junction of the anterior and middle cranial fossae is located at the apex of the orbit.

Symptoms and signs of orbital disease

Orbital diseases often cause displacement of the eyeball. Protrusion is called proptosis or exophthalmos. If the volume of the orbital contents is increased, expansion can occur only anteriorly provided the walls of the orbit are intact, and so proptosis or exophthalmos is the main clinical indicator of orbital disease.

Proptosis, especially if it is unilateral, is best appreciated by standing behind and above the patient and looking down the vertical plane of the patient's face. More sophisticated ways of recognizing proptosis are available but the above method suffices.

Examples of mistaken diagnoses of proptosis (especially unilateral) are the large eyeball in myopia (*see* Plate 13.1), asymmetry of the eyelids and orbits, or enophthalmos (sunken eye) on the *other* side. Upper lid retraction may also simulate proptosis but the latter is probably not present if the observer, looking at the patient from the front, sees the margin of the *lower* lid 'touch' the limbus (=corneoscleral junction). If the two are separated by a gap, with white sclera showing, proptosis is more likely.

It is important to decide whether the proptosis is axial (i.e. the eyeball being pushed forwards) or non-axial (the eyeball being pushed forwards but to one side or upwards or downwards) because this will help to decide where the lesion lies in the orbit. It is important to ask the patient about the onset, duration and course of the symptoms, as these factors may help to elucidate the pathology of the lesion (Table 13.1).

RAPID ONSET	Adults	Ophthalmic Graves' disease
		Orbital cellulitis
		Pseudotumours
	Children	Orbital cellulitis
		Rhabdomyosarcoma
		Metastatic disease
		(neuroblastoma, leukaemias)
SLOW ONSET		Dermoid cyst
		Mixed lacrimal gland tumour
		Cavernous haemangioma

Table 13.1 Common causes of proptosis and type of onset

Proptosis may be associated with other signs such as decreased visual acuity, double vision, ptosis or lid retraction, congestion and oedema of the eyelids and conjunctiva. In some conditions the patient may complain of pain, for example, in orbital cellulitis or orbital haemorrhage.

Diagnosis and investigation of proptosis

A full history must be taken. Inspection of old photographs for comparison is often valuable. Consideration must be given to sinus disease, nasopharyngeal and intracranial disease, especially tumours. Tests for thyroid disease and tests to exclude haemopoietic disorders are often important. X-ray of the orbits and optic foramina, including tomography, may be required.

Computer-assisted tomography (CAT) scanning has revolutionized

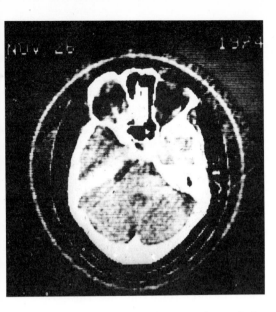

Fig 13.1 CAT scan showing thickening of the extraocular muscles in thyroid eye disease.

the investigation of orbital disease. This radiological technique can locate many orbital masses in both the sagittal and the coronal planes, and may show features which indicate the precise pathological diagnosis (Fig 13.1). Carotid angiography has been used frequently in the past to delineate orbital vascular lesions but a new development—much less hazardous and less invasive, using computing techniques, namely digital vascular imaging—is becoming available and its place in the investigation of the orbit is assured. Ultrasound scanning is also used in the investigation of orbital conditions; B-scanning gives a view of the orbit which delineates the location and size of the orbital lesion while an A-scan may lead to tissue diagnosis because of specific patterns of echoes which different lesions make. Nuclear magnetic resonance (NMR), even less invasive than CAT scanning, will probably improve diagnostic methods further.

Causes of orbital disease

Below is a list, in order of frequency, of common orbital disorders in adults. The first on the list is very, very much the most common.

Ophthalmic Graves' disease
Pseudotumour
Direct extension of tumours from neighbouring sites
Metastatic tumours—mainly breast and lung
Cavernous haemangioma

Lacrimal gland tumours
Lymphoma
Meningioma
Mucocele from a neighbouring sinus
Dermoid cyst
Orbital cellulitis

In children the commonest cause of proptosis is orbital cellulitis as a complication of ethmoid sinusitis or respiratory infection. Dermoids and capillary haemangiomata are the most common benign orbital childhood tumours while rhabdomyosarcomata are the most common primary orbital malignant childhood tumours.

Thyroid eye disease

This is the commonest cause of orbital disease in adults, females being affected eight times more often than males. Most of the signs are caused by an increase in the volume of the intraorbital contents. The most important signs are upper lid retraction due to sympathetic overstimulation (*see* Plate 13.2), upper lid lag on down-gaze, unilateral or bilateral exophthalmos, diplopia, oedema of eyelids and conjunctivae, injection over the horizontal muscle insertions and, rarely, corneal exposure due to inability of the lids to provide adequate protection for the protruded eyeball and/or visual failure due to optic nerve compression (*see* Plate 13.3).

The extraocular muscles may swell up to eight times their normal size, and waterlogging of orbital fat occurs. These changes are secondary to an antigen–antibody reaction in the orbit where connective tissue is the antigen and, probably, a subunit of the thyroid-stimulating hormone (TSH) molecule is the antibody. *These patients MAY not show any of the other classic signs of thyroid disease*, but must be investigated fully in this regard—thyroxine levels, TSH levels, tri-iodothyronine and antithyroid antibody levels to name but a few. In most cases little treatment is required; topical lubricants such as methylcellulose eyedrops, and occasionally 5% guanethidine eyedrops to relieve lid retraction, may suffice. If periorbital oedema is marked a mild diuretic may help, but if the proptosis is severe and vision is threatened (1% of cases) systemic steroid therapy (up to 80 mg prednisone per day) must be used. This can be augmented by azathioprine 100 mg per day until the proptosis begins to resolve. Surgical decompression of the orbits by removal of the orbital floors may be necessary in very severe cases. Diplopia can be treated by prisms initially but when the condition has been stable for at least one year, operation on the extraocular muscles may be considered.

Orbital inflammation

Most acute orbital inflammations originate from the adjacent sinuses, in particular the ethmoid sinuses. A cellulitis may arise from rupture of an infected sinus into the orbit or as an extension by thrombophlebitis. There is severe swelling of the lids and conjunctiva, and eye movements are usually very restricted (*see* Plate 13.4). There is severe pain, and the patient is constitutionally ill with fever and malaise. If a collection of pus is observed it should be drained (e.g. an infected nasal sinus or an orbital abscess), and systemic antibiotic treatment is essential to prevent the spread of the infection intracranially.

The commonest chronic inflammation of the orbit is a chronic granuloma called a *pseudotumour*. These pseudotumours are mainly non-specific inflammatory reactions and histologically are composed of fibroblasts, many eosinophils and perivascular lymphocytic infiltrations. Middle-aged men are predominantly involved and the onset is usually acute with rapid development of proptosis, diplopia and pain. Systemic steroid therapy, up to 60 mg prednisone per day, is often diagnostic in that resolution of the condition occurs on such therapy.

Cavernous sinus thrombosis is an acute thrombophlebitis originating from an infected area which has venous drainage to the cavernous sinus. *The patient is severely ill* with fever and malaise, and eventually may develop meningitis. Proptosis and chemosis (oedema of conjunctiva) start usually in one eye but become bilateral within a day or two, while pain in the ophthalmic division of the trigeminal nerve is common. Prompt and effective systemic antibiotic treatment is necessary if meningitis and intracranial abscess are to be prevented.

Orbital trauma

Blunt trauma

The commonest result of blunt orbital trauma is an orbital haematoma (black eye). This may be painful, and once a reduction in the swelling of the lids has occurred the visual acuity of the involved eye should be checked and the fundus examined to exclude intraocular contusion. Severe intraorbital haemorrhage may also be a sign of a fracture of an orbital wall.

A marked increase in intraorbital pressure may cause a *blow-out fracture* of the orbital floor, with herniation of orbital contents into the maxillary sinus which can be seen on x-ray tomographs of the orbital floor. Another suggested mechanism is a blow on the malar bone, which transmits fracturing force to the orbital floor. Diplopia on looking up results; if necessary an exploratory operation to free the trapped tissue should be carried out within two weeks of the injury.

Fractures of the orbital margins often occur in facial fractures and should always be looked for in severe facial injury. Careful palpation, especially along the malar arch, is important because a radiograph may be difficult to interpret; the clinician is looking for bony crepitus and subcutaneous emphysema indicating involvement of an air sinus.

Penetrating orbital injury

After a penetrating wound of the orbit, there should always be a high index of suspicion that a foreign body may be embedded in the orbit. X-ray studies should be done, and if the intraorbital foreign body is small and metallic it is probably best left alone—particularly if it is in the posterior orbit (Fig 13.2). If, however, vegetable matter has become

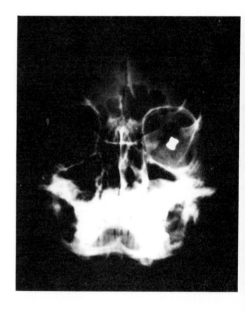

Fig 13.2 Intraorbital foreign body (airgun pellet).

lodged in the orbit (e.g. a twig or leaves from a tree), the wound should be explored as far as possible and all vegetable matter removed; if this is not done, chronic or acute relapsing inflammation will occur with proptosis and the possibility of intracranial spread.

Further reading

Henderson J W (1973) *Orbital Tumors*. Philadelphia: W B Saunders
Krohel G B, Stewart W B and Chavis R M (1981) *Orbital Disease*. New York: Grune & Stratton
Newell F W and Ernest J T (1982) *Ophthalmology*. St Louis: C V Mosby
Spaeth G L (ed) (1982) *Ophthalmic Surgery*. Philadelphia: W B Saunders

14

The Dry or Watering Eye

P A Hunter

The dry eye

The normal tear film

The presence of a normal precorneal (or, more accurately, preocular) tear film is important for several reasons. Chief of these is that it provides for a smooth optical interface at the front surface of the eye by bridging minute irregularities in the surface epithelium. It lubricates the movement of the eyelids and has important protective functions in that foreign matter can be removed by irrigation and the aqueous component contains lysozymes, IgG and secretory IgA, which assist in the defence against micro-organisms. Desquamated corneal epithelial cells are also eliminated by the constant irrigation.

The stability of the tear film is dependent on the presence of three components, together with a number of other factors (Fig 14.1). The outermost portion consists of waxy and cholesterol esters which are fluid at body temperature and are derived from the meibomian glands in the eyelids. By forming a monolayer on the surface they are said to help retain the aqueous layer by their surface tension properties and help

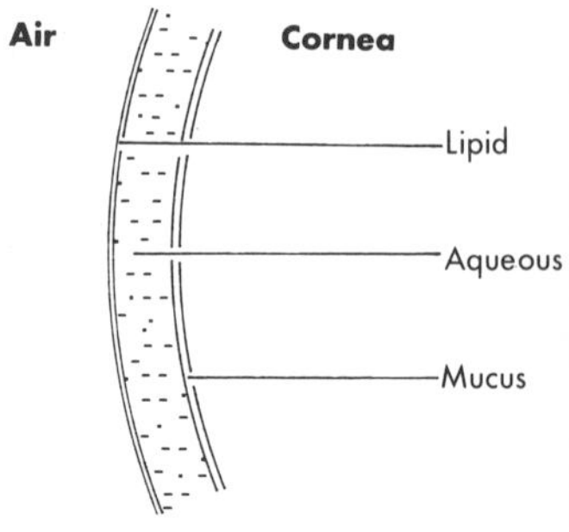

Fig 14.1 The normal tear film.

reduce evaporation. The aqueous layer is secreted by the main and accessory lacrimal glands, and account for 90% of the thickness of the normal tear film. Between the aqueous layer and the corneal epithelial surface a thin layer of mucus is interposed. The molecular structure of the mucus component is polarized so that one end of the molecule is hydrophilic and the other hydrophobic, and the molecules are so arranged that they interact with the aqueous layer and phospholipid cell membrane of the epithelium respectively. In this way, 'wetting' of the corneal epithelium is achieved by the mucus which is derived from the goblet cells found mainly in the conjunctival fornices. The normal tear film, therefore, derives elements from the lids, conjunctiva and lacrimal glands. In addition, a normal blink reflex is required to allow regeneration and circulation of the tears to take place.

The abnormal tear film

If the tear film components or blinking are defective in quantity or quality, 'drying' of all or part of the surface of the eye takes place, resulting in a wide range of pathology. In its mildest form this consists of a sensation variously described as grittiness, dryness or irritation, and is usually accompanied by punctate staining of the lower half of the cornea and conjunctiva (keratoconjunctivitis sicca). More severe forms show signs of conjunctival inflammation and the integrity of the epithelium may be jeopardized. Small erosions may enlarge, or filaments consisting of mucus and epithelial débris attach themselves to damaged areas (filamentary keratitis; *see* Plate 14.1). Frank corneal ulceration may be complicated by secondary bacterial infection leading to endophthalmitis. Although this last complication is fortunately rare, it is the main pathway to blindness in those areas of the world where vitamin A deficiency causing xerophthalmia leads to a high prevalence of keratomalacia.

The pathogenesis of these diseases is probably best reflected in the concept of a 'non-wetting' ocular surface rather than the term 'dry eye' which implies merely a reduction in the aqueous component of the tears. Thus the symptoms and signs already described may be the product of, for example, insufficient mucus production which may occur in the presence of normal or even excessive watery secretion when the term 'dry' would hardly seem to be appropriate. The concept of non-wetting of the eye should alert the physician to examine all aspects of the tear film and hence ensure that the correct remedy is chosen.

Investigation

For reasons already explained the examination of the poorly wetting eye should include the whole of the external eye and adnexae, not merely the cornea. An approximate estimate of volume of the aqueous component can be made by studying the meniscus of tears that forms along the lower lid margin where it makes contact with the globe. Schirmer's test has been advocated as a measure of tear production. In this test, a strip of filter paper 5 × 35 mm is folded at one end which is then placed with the short end in the lower conjunctival fornix. The amount of wetting that occurs in the protruding long end is measured after a period of one minute. Unfortunately, the test is poorly reproducible in a single patient and the measurements so obtained are unreliable as a basis of a quantitative test. It does, however, offer an indication as to which patients are 'very dry' and may therefore enable guidelines to be given as to what frequency of artificial tear supplements should be used in therapy. As yet, there are no methods of quantifying meibomian or mucus secretion. The relative quantities of these components can only be inferred by observing the 'break-up time' of the precorneal tear film.

In this test, the eyelids are held apart and, following staining with fluorescein, the precorneal tear film is studied using the slit-lamp. The time taken for dry spots to appear is noted. As with Schirmer's test, absolute measurements are unreliable but if break-up time occurs within a few seconds, an imbalance (either excess or lack) of either meibomian or mucus secretion should be suspected.

Abnormalities of meibomian secretion

From a practical standpoint, inadequate meibomian secretion does not occur. Tear film abnormalities may, however, result from excessive production which is often seen clinically as frothy tears. This is nearly always caused by chronic meibomian gland infection (meibomitis) in chronic blepharitis or acne rosacea. Treatment consists of controlling the underlying lid disease, which usually involves long-term therapy.

Diminished lacrimal secretion

Reduced lacrimal secretion is undoubtedly most frequently seen as part of the involutional change occurring with age, commonly starting with the menopause in females. Lacrimal gland involvement is a not infrequent complication of a variety of systemic disorders which include rheumatoid arthritis and sarcoidosis. Sjögren's syndrome consists of reduced lacrimal and salivary secretion occurring in 15% of patients with rheumatoid arthritis. The other ocular signs of sarcoid include conjunctival and iris nodules, uveitis and retinal vasculitis: if these are seen, further investigation of the patient is indicated. An extremely rare cause of reduced lacrimal secretion is familial dysautonomia (Riley–Day syndrome) which is seen only in Jewish populations.

Treatment of all these conditions is primarily symptomatic based on artificial tear supplements. The simplest of such preparations would be normal saline drops, but their effect is so transient that more viscous preparations such as methylcellulose or hydroxypropyl methylcellulose (hypromellose) are usually employed. Treatment dosages are determined by the patient who may use them as little or as often as the symptoms dictate. In severe cases, occlusion of the lacrimal puncta may be carried out.

Abnormalities of mucus secretion

This is usually the result of conjunctival scarring which gives rise to diminished secretion from damaged goblet cells. The causes include trachoma, chemical burns and autoimmune diseases such as Stevens–Johnson syndrome and benign mucous membrane pemphigoid. Although symptomatic relief may be obtained through artificial tears, it may be more logical to use mucomimetic agents such as polyvinylpyrrolidone to promote surface wetting, rather than increase the tear volume which may already be sufficient.

The watering eye

Epiphora is the overflow of tears onto the cheek due to excessive tear secretion or diminished tear drainage. Where it is of pathological significance, excessive tear secretion is almost invariably reflexly produced as a result of corneal or conjunctival irritation. In such cases, additional symptoms and signs will usually indicate a treatable cause, the management of which has already been discussed (Chapter 6). Where watering alone is a symptom, a cause is often to be found in defective lacrimal drainage, and careful examination and investigation are then required to determine the most appropriate treatment.

The normal lacrimal drainage system (Fig 14.2)

The tears enter the lacrimal drainage system via the lacrimal puncta which are situated at the medial ends of the upper and lower eyelids. Normal blinking assists in the movement of tears medially where they enter the upper and lower canaliculi and, later, the lacrimal sac. It is probable that, during lid closure, deep fibres of the orbicularis oculi muscle distend the lacrimal sac and draw fluid into it by a lacrimal pump mechanism. Almost

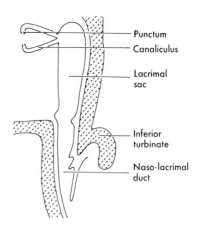

Fig 14.2 Diagram of a coronal section of the right lacrimal drainage system.

Punctum
Canaliculus
Lacrimal sac
Inferior turbinate
Naso-lacrimal duct

equal quantities of tears flow through the upper and lower canaliculi and the system does not appear to work on a 'gravity feed' principle, as was once thought, with the majority of the tears flowing via the inferior canaliculus. From the lacrimal sac, drainage is via the nasolacrimal duct into the lateral wall of the nose where it opens in the inferior meatus. The nasolacrimal duct lies within a bony canal with a series of incomplete valve-like membranes within its lumen.

Defective lacrimal drainage

Pathological conditions anywhere along the drainage system (Fig 14.2) may produce epiphora. Absent or impaired blinking such as occurs in a lower motor neuron palsy of the VIIth nerve impairs the normal pumping mechanism of the sac. Tears may fail to gain access to the puncta due to their malposition (ectropion) or stenosis. Canalicular blockage due to trauma or chronic infection and nasolacrimal duct obstruction (either congenital or acquired) both produce epiphora, which may be accompanied by the presence of a mucocele (*see* Plate 14.2). If a mucocele becomes secondarily infected, it presents as a tender red swelling immediately below the medial canthus (acute dacryocystitis), when it requires treatment with systemic antibiotics and subsequent drainage surgery to prevent recurrence. Finally, the obstruction may lie within the nasal passages, in which situation it may all too easily be overlooked by the unwary ophthalmologist. The localization of the site of obstruction is mandatory if the appropriate treatment is to be given.

Investigation

A careful history and examination are an essential prerequisite of any investigation of epiphora. Enquiries in the history should be directed towards past inflammatory ocular disease, trauma, the use of medications and previous nasal problems, and the examiner should then exclude hypersecretion of tears before noting any abnormality in blinking, evidence of ectropion and the state of the puncta. Thereafter, investigation may require more invasive techniques and it is important to realize the potential for inducing further damage before embarking on such procedures.

The injection of saline solution into one or other puncta (syringing) is used as a method of testing the anatomical integrity of the lacrimal passages at and below the level of the common canaliculus. If fluid passes freely into the nasopharynx, the nasolacrimal duct is said to be patent— although it should be remembered that such a test is not physiological. If fluid regurgitates through the other punctum, together with the mucous contents of the lacrimal sac, the blockage is deemed to lie in the nasolacrimal duct. If clear fluid without mucus regurgitates and, furthermore, regurgitation does not take place when gentle pressure is exerted over the lacrimal sac, the block is at the opening of the common canaliculus into the sac. At this stage sufficient information should be available to enable an accurate diagnosis to be made. Occasionally, further investigations may be required; these include dacrocystography using radio-opaque contrast media or lacrimal scintillography with radioactively labelled sodium pertechnate.

Probing the lacrimal canaliculi may demonstrate a blockage proximal to the sac and, by measuring the length of probe admitted, its site can be accurately determined.

Treatment

The treatment of the commoner causes of epiphora is outlined below.

Ectropion
Surgical correction is indicated in the majority of cases where epiphora is a problem (Chapter 12). Minor degrees may be corrected using retropunctal cautery.

Punctal stenosis
This is usually acquired as a result of chronic inflammatory disease leading to scarring. Such cases may be helped surgically by marsupializing part of the canaliculus using a 'three-snip procedure'. Punctal stenosis may also arise through the long-term use of topical antiviral agents such as idoxuridine which, if recognized early enough, is reversible on stopping the drug.

Canalicular blockage

This is the most difficult to treat satisfactorily. An acute infection (canaliculitis) due to streptothrix will be cured by marsupialization and topical penicillin drops. However, in chronic infections (e.g. trachoma, herpes simplex) scarring of the canaliculi can be treated only by the insertion of a glass tube (Lester Jones tube) directly from the conjunctiva to the nose. If sufficient normal canaliculus is present, the canaliculi can be anastomosed directly to the nasal mucosa (canaliculodacryocystorhinostomy, CDCR) but the results of this operation are variable.

Common canalicular blockage

This may be due to canalicular stenosis (when a CDCR may help) or a mucosal thickening around its opening into the sac. In the case of the latter, anastomosis of the lacrimal sac mucosa to the nasal mucosa via a rhinostomy (dacrocystorhinostomy, DCR) enables any distal blockage to be circumvented whilst temporary polythene tubes are inserted via the canaliculi into the nose through the rhinostomy. These maintain the integrity of the common canalicular opening while healing occurs (DCR and tubes).

Nasolacrimal duct blockage

This may be congenital or acquired in later life. Congenital obstruction is due to delay in the normal development of the system and is present in 2–4% of all infants at birth. The majority of these will eventually canalize normally during the first six months of life, and conservative treatment using antibiotic drops if the eye is sticky, coupled with expression of the sac, is all that is required. If full canalization of the nasolacrimal duct does not occur, a simple probing under anaesthetic will alleviate the problem. Acquired blockage of the duct is treated surgically if the symptoms are sufficiently troublesome, in which case a dacrocystorhinostomy (DCR) is performed. Although the operation when carried out correctly has an almost 100% success rate, it is often well worth reassuring the patient with epiphora that the watering is not harmful to the eye, which may well spare both doctor and patient the rigours of surgery.

15 Tropical Ophthalmology

Blinding xerophthalmia and keratomalacia: vitamin A deficiency J D C Anderson

'Doctors know that . . . green vegetables, even leaves, make all the difference between vision and blindness. But rural people and many in the cities are still unaware of such elementary facts.' Indira Gandhi (1976)

Deficiency of vitamin A, which is easily preventable, blinds more than a quarter of a million children in the world every year, especially in Asia.

Clinical features

Retina

The first symptom is usually greater difficulty than normal in seeing in dull illumination ('night blindness') because of poor dark adaptation due to defective visual purple in the rods of the retina; ingested vitamin A (= retinol) is essential for maintenance of visual purple. Little children of course cannot verbalize this symptom but their mothers notice they are blind after dusk, hence the often used local phrase 'chicken-eyes' for night blindness. (Chicken eyes have only cones with no rods hence their night blindness.)

Conjunctiva and cornea

The next stage is bilateral *dryness* of the conjunctiva and cornea (xerophthalmia), with loss of mucus-producing goblet cells and conversion of epithelia into a stratified squamous form with keratinization—i.e. the mucous membrane becomes skin-like. An early sign is Bitot's spots, which are triangular patches of conjunctiva, on each side of the cornea, covered with foamy or cheesy material: they are often pigmented and may remain after vitamin A deficiency has disappeared.

Under adverse conditions, such as continued severe malnutrition or an attack of diarrhoea or measles, this may be followed acutely by melting away of both corneae (keratomalacia), until perforation occurs.

Perforation of the cornea causes escape of aqueous humour, and flattening of the anterior chamber: the iris usually plugs the gap and the anterior chamber re-forms, leaving part of the iris adherent to the cornea (anterior synechia). A large area of the cornea may be converted to white scar tissue or 'leukoma'. In severe cases, because of large corneal perforations, the eye may collapse entirely and never re-fill with aqueous humour; the globe remains a small shrunken mass in the orbit, a condition called phthisis bulbi (or 'wasting of the globe'). Other deficiencies nearly always coexist, especially protein-energy malnutrition, which predispose to infections. These in turn aggravate the diseases due to deficiency, as the following case history shows (*see* Plate 15.1).

CASE HISTORY

Abdi Aden Gulet was the second of four boys in a poor Somali family. At the age of 3 years he became acutely ill because of measles which mopped up his little remaining vitamin A (he was already night blind) so that severe bilateral keratomalacia developed. He nearly died. Now, aged 15 years, his right eye has a heavily scarred cornea giving only 'perception of light', while the left eyeball is completely shrunken. He has no alternative but to beg for a living (*see* Plate 15.1).

Treatment should be given urgently: 200 000 IU of vitamin A by mouth on two successive days, but if there is severe gastroenteritis or protein deficiency, an intramuscular injection of 100 000 IU of **watermiscible** vitamin A could be given followed by oral vitamin A after 24 hours. A protein-rich and calorie-rich diet should be given, and any systemic infection treated. The minimum local eye treatment should ideally be a prophylactic antibiotic eye ointment three times daily. The mothers of marasmic infants should be taught to use their fingers to close their children's eyelids gently, and repeatedly, whenever necessary. (In Western countries where head injuries, facial paralysis and general anaesthesia are the common causes of corneal exposure, adhesive tape is usually easily available to apply to the upper lids to pull them down towards the cheeks, if an antibiotic eye ointment (i.e. oculentum) will not suffice.)

Prevention has supreme importance, and in places where this disease occurs it is primary health care workers who hold the key to effective prevention. They must be taught to **identify the children at risk.** They must become aware of the vulnerable age group, learn to recognize the malnourished ones (i.e. those with a mid-arm circumference of 12.5 cm or less—at any age), and be taught how to encourage the home-growing and eating of dark green leafy vegetables and yellow fruits—all rich in beta-carotene, the precursor of vitamin A; they can also give oral vitamin A to vulnerable children and be instructed in the effective oral rehydration treatment of diarrhoea. It is they who can best influence families to accept measles vaccination or to give sensible home care to children who have contracted it. Primary health care workers are crucial to any effective strategy for prevention.

Other current preventive measures are the twice-yearly oral administration of vitamin A (200 000 IU) to the 1- to 5-year-old age group, or the fortification of a universally consumed food such as sugar or tea with a stable and tasteless form of vitamin A. Additional preventive measures reduce the prevalence of infection; for example, safe water to control diarrhoea, or immunization against measles, pertussis and tuberculosis.

At a more fundamental level, the problems of poverty, malnutrition and infection remain.

Trachoma   J D C Anderson

Trachoma is the world's most serious cause of poor vision, affecting about 500 million people of whom 100 million suffer some visual handicap and at least 2 million are totally blind.

The most important feature of this chronic and recurrent inflammation of conjunctiva and cornea, due to infection by *Chlamydia trachomatis*, is the frequent and often serious results of scar formation (cicatrization) in these tissues and in the eyelids.

The *C. trachomatis* is a minute atypical bacterium, which divides by binary fission, though it grows only inside certain epithelial cells. It has a cell wall, contains both DNA and RNA (viruses contain only DNA *or* RNA), and has a limited enzyme system. Like bacteria, it is sensitive to sulphonamides and to some antibiotics. From a dozen or more serotypes detected by the microimmunofluorescence test, most of which are found in genital and other extraocular infections, only three are regularly found in endemic trachoma associated with eye-to-eye transmission.

This infective agent invades the non-keratinized epithelial cells of the conjunctiva and cornea as rigid-walled elementary bodies 300 nm in diameter. After 48 hours, these have multiplied themselves by upwards of a thousandfold and form intracytoplasmic inclusion bodies adjacent to the nuclei of the epithelial cells. These inclusions can be seen in iodine- or Giemsa-stained conjunctival smears. The host cell then ruptures and thousands of elementary bodies are freed to invade more epithelial cells.

Although these bodies may not themselves invade the subepithelial tissues, their toxic metabolic products almost certainly do, and these induce an inflammatory reaction in the cornea, conjunctiva and adjacent tissues. The degree of inflammation and subsequent scarring in trachoma is determined by a combination of factors: first, the total period of time (months or, more likely, years) in which the individual has been repeatedly reinfected; secondly , the dose of Chlamydia introduced at each reinfection; and thirdly, the amount of eye damage sustained from other causes, such as bacterial and viral infections or trauma. Prolonged and rather ineffective immune responses are responsible both for the disastrous scarring of cornea and eyelids in trachoma and for the resultant physical signs.

Epidemiology

The documented history of this disease dates back to 2500 BC. Today it occurs in the 'trachoma belt'—North Africa, the Middle East, the Indian subcontinent and the Far East—but it is also found in parts of southern Europe, in Central and Latin America and amongst the aboriginal people of Australia. Important factors encouraging its maintenance and spread in a population are overcrowding and poor water supply, each contributing to insanitary conditions; for example, shared water for washing, common cloths for drying and absence of latrines. But an additional and escalating factor in the spread and maintenance of trachoma is the frequently high prevalence of 'eye-seeking' flies (see Plate 15.2)—particularly the common housefly and the smaller *Musca sorbens* which grows preferentially on human faeces. These flies, needing moisture and protein (to mature their eggs), move from exposed faeces to the watering eyes and discharging noses of different individuals indiscriminately. They have been proved to be carriers of both bacteria *and* Chlamydia [1], which explains why the 'fly season' is followed so closely by the 'sticky eye season'. Epidemics of mucopurulent *bacterial* conjunctivitis usually occur during the fly season and so, indirectly, enhance reinfection with *Chlamydia trachomatis* because the flies are not selective in what they transport from the eyes of one person to another! Only in recent years has the importance of *multiple* reinfection with Chlamydia, especially if combined with bacterial infection, been recognized as the major factor in the development of severe scarring in trachoma. In this complex process of reinfection, flies appear to have a significant role.

In the UK 150 years ago trachoma was a serious public health problem. But 50 years before antibiotics were ever discovered it had vanished with the advent of laws on housing, piped water, improved sewage disposal and better hygiene.

The classic *stages of trachoma* described by MacCallan are useful for identifying four moderately well-defined points in the pathogenesis of a first infection. But their value is limited for two reasons: first, because they are based primarily on the conjunctival signs; and secondly, because we now recognize that trachoma is a multicyclic infection and so the very same conjunctival membrane may show, for example, the scarring of stage III in one location *and* some early follicles of stage I in another. Hence, this classification by stages has no real prognostic value. MacCallan's classification is here summarized:

Stage I   *Incipient trachoma*: immature follicles on upper tarsal conjunctiva; early corneal signs present.

Stage II   *Established trachoma*: well-developed follicles on tarsal plates; papillary hypertrophy and diffuse infiltration. Corneal pannus extending from upper limbus (*see* Plate 15.3); limbal follicles or even Herbert's pits.

Stage III   *Cicatrizing trachoma*: all the above signs plus conjunctival scarring (*see* Plate 15.4).

Stage IV   *Healed trachoma*: all inflammation has subsided; the eye is no longer infectious; but scars remain for life and further damage may occur as a result.

Symptoms

Symptoms of trachoma in the early stages range from almost nil to a mild bilateral ocular discomfort with a little watering, or to a severe foreign body sensation with marked photophobia. If secondary bacterial infection is present there may be redness of the eyes, discharge and crusting of the lid margins. In advanced trachoma with severe scarring, patients may complain of heaviness of the eyelids, foreign body sensation and blurring of vision. If their eyelashes are turned inwards (trichiasis) the irritation and watering are constant (*see* Plate 15.5). Extensive scarring makes the eyes feel dry. However, the majority of trachoma subjects in fact complain of few symptoms. Millions of others learn to live with their progressive trachoma uncomplainingly.

Signs

Conjunctival early signs are best seen (with the help of torch and magnifying loupe) on the everted lids, especially the upper lids. Here, particularly in the fornices and over the upper tarsal plate, lymphoid *follicles* can be seen; i.e. little (0.2–2 mm diameter), yellowish-white, raised, avascular lesions which vary from few to numerous. After weeks or months, these small lesions may, in severe infections, become large, yellow and necrotic, and be partially buried in thickened conjunctiva. They represent a cell-mediated specific immune response to the infective agent. The conjunctival membrane becomes thickened by a diffuse cellular infiltration (of neutrophils, lymphocytes, plasma cells, macrophages) and by neovascularization. This produces two very important signs: first, the appearance of multiple tiny engorged capillary tufts, called *papillae*, on the surface of the conjunctiva, which, when numerous, give it a red velvety appearance; and secondly, a partial or even complete obscuration of the normally visible conjunctival blood vessels (*see* Plate 15.2–15.7). This latter sign indicates a very severe inflammatory reaction. As the disease develops, small linear scars or, in more severe cases, large confluent scars appear after some months and are a permanent record of this disease. These scars contract and in so doing may produce serious complications.

Corneal early signs appear first and foremost in its upper half—a fact which is related to the cornea's close contact with the upper lid. In order to see that area, obviously the upper lid has to be held up. Lesions are so small at first as to require a magnifying loupe or slit-lamp microscope to be seen. In long-standing trachoma the whole cornea may become affected. Epithelial keratitis with tiny shallow ulcers (shown up well with fluorescein staining) is followed by cellular infiltration of the stroma under the infected epithelium. It is then that the fibrovascular membrane, known as trachomatous *pannus* (Latin, 'cloth'), begins to invade the superficial stroma (*see* Plate 15.3). Follicles are sometimes prominent at the upper limbal region of the cornea. When these heal, they leave shallow translucent depressions called *Herbert's pits*, which are pathognomonic of trachoma.

External lid signs may be entirely absent. However, some degree of lid swelling often reflects a more severe tarsal infection. It settles with healing. With the scarring of long-standing trachoma, the lids may become thickened and in-turned (entropion); a few or many lashes may rub against the cornea (trichiasis, *see* Plate 15.5); the lid aperture may be abnormally widened from scarring of the lid retractors, or the lid margins may become notched from scarring. In consequence there may be a defect in lid closure which is noticed when the patient blinks or is asked to close his eyes gently as in sleep.

Complications

These are all a direct or indirect result of scarring. In the *cornea*, scarring causes blurring of vision indirectly by distorting the corneal curvature and directly by causing central corneal opacities. The cornea's resistance to secondary infection is compromised by two factors: first, the constant trauma from the in-turned lashes of trichiasis; and secondly, from inadequate wetting by tears. This latter problem results partly from failure of the scarred up conjunctival goblet cells to produce mucin and partly from blockage of the tear ducts but also often from sheer mechanical failure of a distorted and contracted eyelid to sweep an even tear film over the cornea. A compromised cornea is always at risk of bacterial or other infection, and so corneal ulceration leading to suppurative keratitis is one of the pathways to blindness in chronic trachoma.

Treatment

Treatment of the individual

Antibiotics rapidly (about 10 days) make an individual Chlamydia-free, because they prevent multiplication of the agent within the epithelial cells which are routinely shed from the surfaces within about 10 days. Where the conjunctiva is severely disorganized, treatment is required for several weeks. The signs may take three months to disappear.

Both of the following, alone or together, are effective:

1 **Oral** sulphonamide (e.g. triple sulpha) for three weeks or a long-acting drug such as sulfametopyrazine (30 mg/kg), one dose per week for three weeks. The risks of sulphonamide complications (e.g. the rare Stevens–Johnson syndrome) must be considered. Alternatively, **oral** tetracycline 250 mq q.i.d., or doxycycline 100 mg daily, for three weeks is effective.
2 **Topical** tetracycline 1% ointment instilled into the conjunctival sac three times daily for six weeks.

Surgical treatment of the lid deformities is necessary for three reasons: first, to reduce the risk of blinding complications such as corneal ulceration; secondly, to relieve the patient's physical discomfort; and thirdly, to make the eye less watery and less attractive to eye-seeking flies. Mild trichiasis is often treated by simple epilation, which must be repeated because the distorted lashes grow again. Electrolysis of individual lashes may succeed in a localized area of trichiasis, but it is difficult and unpleasant. Cryotherapy is a more satisfactory method. Many useful operations have been devised to correct cicatricial entropion of the upper and lower eyelids. Great vigilance is required to diagnose exposure keratitis, which needs careful treatment. Finally, corneal grafting is often disappointing in trachoma: because of the difficulty in maintaining good after-care with topical corticosteroid immunosuppressives, host–graft reaction in the inhospitable vascularized host cornea may cause the graft to become opaque.

Treatment of the community

The immediate aim here is different from that in the individual, because the problem is different. The problem in a community with hyperendemic trachoma is the continuing pressure of transmission of infection from the **ocular community pool** of *Chlamydia trachomatis* constantly being topped up by multiple infected persons, especially children, who reinfect each other and make individual treatment disappointing (*see* Plates 15.6 and 15.7). Emphasis must be placed on ways of breaking the cycles of reinfection and of reducing the community concentration of Chlamydia. Just as venereal disease could be eliminated by reducing promiscuity, so trachoma could be eliminated or reduced to safe levels by attacking transmission points. The most important preventive measures are listed below:

1   provide a plentiful water supply (e.g. by well-digging);
2   give health education to the community, especially school children, about the disease and its spread;
3   introduce fly-control measures; and, related to that—
4   encourage the provision and clean use of latrines;
5   increase the birth interval by family-planning to reduce the population-density of small children living close together, who collect, multiply and shed Chlamydia to others.
6   *ideally* provide more spacious housing! But how?
7   provide drug treatment on a mass scale to all children under 10 years of age but especially to the preschool children, in order to reduce the ocular reservoir of Chlamydia in the community. One regimen recommended by the World Health Organization is to give tetracycline ointment to school children as follows: twice daily every day for **one** week in every month for **six** months. There are several other, equally effective, regimens.

In a Somali refugee camp of 60 000 people a survey indicated a high prevalence of active trachoma, described as a 'forest fire'. A simple programme was carried out by 15 refugee community health workers and one Somali nurse. They combined a face- and hand-washing programme among school and preschool children with a once daily instillation of 3% tetracycline ointment. Some fly control was also attempted. The result was impressive. A second survey showed a reduction of active trachoma to **one-third** of its previous level.

The lesson? **Blinding trachoma** is a **community problem** that could be rapidly controlled by highly motivated community action.

1 Jones B R (1975) The prevention of blindness from trachoma. *Trans Ophthalmol Soc UK* **95**, 16–33

Onchocerciasis M G Kerr-Muir

This is a blinding disease caused by the filarial worm *Onchocerca volvulus*, transmitted by the blackfly (Simulium species), occurring in Central and South America, equatorial Africa and the Yemen. Blindness results from involvement of the optic nerve, chorioretina and cornea, and from glaucoma and cataract secondary to long-standing iritis.

Epidemiology

Of the estimated 50 million infected persons, one million are blind, with many more severely disabled, the incidence of blindness being related to the microfilarial load, which in turn depends on the intensity and duration of transmission. The devastation for the individual is compounded for the community because the blindness affects the young working population, and the voracious biting habit of the flies, in addition to their capacity as vectors, has rendered many fertile riverine areas uninhabitable.

Man is the definitive host and reservoir of this microfilarial load produced continually by adult female worms which can survive for up to 15 years in the human body. These microfilariae reside principally in the skin, but also occur in the kidneys, blood and cerebrospinal fluid.

During a blood-meal of the female blackfly, microfilariae gain access to this intermediate host, where they continue their development, and thus disease patterns depend on Simulium behaviour; one important characteristic is its need for well-oxygenated running water at its breeding sites, which thus provide a reasonably circumscribed area for vector control programmes.

Clinical features

Several years usually elapse before the disease becomes manifest, most obviously in the skin as a chronic pruritic eruption leading to atrophy, depigmentation and loss of elasticity, and as subcutaneous nodules which represent coiled masses of adult worms, but the overriding morbidity relates to the ocular consequences of microfilarial infestation.

Microfilariae have been identified histologically in all ocular tissues, and clinically may be seen with a slit-lamp microscope in the cornea, anterior chamber (where the numbers can be dramatically increased by rubbing the eyes or putting the head between the legs for a time prior to examination), and the vitreous.

Examination of conjunctival and skin biopsies shows numerous motile microfilariae, which provide a route of entry to the eye, but it is likely that they also enter along the posterior ciliary vessels and nerves, blood stream and possibly the cerebrospinal fluid.

Where man is a normal host for a parasite, the antibodies formed serve no protective purpose—the parasite has developed tolerance, resulting in a relatively happy host–parasite relationship. However, death of the parasite (or release of its antigens) whether natural or due to drugs, generates a localized inflammatory response which often damages the host tissues. The pattern of disease in onchocerciasis then is related to parasite death and the host's immune response.

Conjunctiva

A mild conjunctivitis occurs, particularly following treatment, and long-standing cases show hyperpigmentation.

Cornea

Typically after early exposure and in mildly infected individuals a localized inflammatory reaction to dead corneal microfilariae leads to a puntate (snowflake) keratitis that usually resolves completely. This represents an immediate hypersensitivity response.

This is in contrast to a characteristic sclerosing keratitis, that only occurs in heavily infected individuals when there is a massive microfilarial load in the inferior cornea, which occurs because there is an impairment of the cell-mediated immunological response. This results in a chronic low-grade inflammatory response with the development of pannus, which progressively opacifies the cornea. It is possible that different parasite strains as well as the variable immunological response contribute to the pattern of clinical disease.

Anterior uvea

An insidious iridocyclitis, often complicated by iris atrophy, posterior synechiae and secondary glaucoma, is an invariable part of the disease and a major contributor to visual impairment. It may be due to microfilariae within the uvea or secondary to corneal disease.

Choroid/Retina (see Plate 15.8)

The morphology of chorioretinal lesions assumes a variety of patterns representing a spectrum of disease from mild pigment epithelial atrophy, that may initially be demonstrable only by fluorescein angiography, through discrete areas of atrophy of retina and underlying choriocapillaris revealing the larger choroidal vessels, to larger areas of atrophy of the posterior pole often with foci of pigment epithelial hyperpigmentation.

Optic nerve

A large proportion of blindness can be attributed to inflammatory disease of the optic nerve, resulting in widespread loss of visual field, compounding the already impaired acuity due to chorioretinal atrophy. Initially, there is a papillitis which resolves into segmental and ultimately total optic atrophy, with corresponding defects in the nerve fibre bundle layer.

Management

Use of the antihelminthic drugs (suramin and diethylcarbamazine) on a community basis is complicated by a high incidence of toxicity affecting the kidney, or the skin as an exfoliative dermatitis or even causing death, and is especially dangerous in those who are heavily infected. In them the aggressive inflammatory reaction, directed against the massive load of dead microfilariae, may make the ocular condition worse. Treatment of individuals with graded or low-dose regimens and anti-inflammatory agents requires careful medical supervision.

Thus, the aim in management is to break the cycle of transmission, and to reduce and eventually remove the human reservoir of microfilariae. This may be achieved by the following.

1 *Decreased exposure to Simulium.* Avoid riverine breeding sites for collection of water by constructing wells and, indeed, villages remote from these areas.
2 *Protective clothing.* Those individuals necessarily exposed to Simulium, such as farmers with running irrigation systems and fishermen, should be encouraged to wear protective clothing.

3 *Nodulectomy.* Skin nodules (containing adult worms), particularly in the head region, should be excised to remove one source of ocular microfilariae.
4 *Insecticides.* The principal method of management of community onchocerciasis is with biodegradable insecticides applied on a regular basis to the riverine breeding sites of Simulium; these must be continued for at least 20 years. The one in common use is temephoss (Abate) manufactured by the American Cyanamid Company, or Cyanamid of Great Britain. The efficacy of this technique demands the co-operation of ophthalmologist, entomologist, parasitologist and epidemiologist in a multidisciplinary approach that also requires a political awareness of the dimensions of the problem to enable continuity of action.

Leprosy   M G Kerr-Muir

Leprosy is a chronic infective disease of neural tissue caused by *Mycobacterium leprae,* a slowly multiplying organism that thrives in a cooler environment so that it preferentially affects superficial tissues. Transmission is principally by droplet spread from the nasal mucosa. It is estimated that 15 million people are affected, of whom about 750 000 are blind. There is a high prevalence in tropical and subtropical areas where overcrowding and poor hygiene are common, especially India and tropical Africa, but climate is not an important limiting factor.

Pathogenesis

An individual's response to exposure to *M. leprae* depends in part upon climate and race but mainly on the type of immunological reaction that follows the initial bacteraemia. There are two main varieties: *tuberculoid,* where there is a brisk cell-mediated response directed at the bacilli *which are rarely found in histological section*; or *lepromatous* (multibacillary) leprosy where the organism multiplies in the absence of an inflammatory reaction, despite the production of humoral antibodies.

Clinical features *(see* Plates 15.9 and 15.10)

There are three distinct pathways to blindness in leprosy, all primarily involving the anterior segment. These are due to:

1 Facial and trigeminal nerve disease
2 Hypersensitivity reaction
3 Direct bacillary invasion of the globe

Diffuse lepromatous disease affects the skin appendages; loss of eyebrows (madarosis) is a common and socially debilitating sequel.

Facial and trigeminal nerve disease

In their superficial course, these nerves are susceptible to leprous invasion, resulting in weakness of the orbicularis oculi muscle (supplied by the seventh cranial nerve) that leads to deficient blinking, inadequate application of the tear film, lower lid ectropion and exposure keratitis. Deficient tear drainage due to ectropion or leprous involvement of the nasolacrimal duct leads to an accumulation of infectious debris, including bacteria and fungi, which may contribute to a suppurative keratitis and rapid disorganization of the cornea. Corneal sensation is impaired due to trigeminal disease, if the patient presents late.

Hypersensitivity reaction

The immune complex hypersensitivity response known as erythema nodosum leprosum, with cutaneous, joint and renal components, is often associated with an acute exudative iritis that may be complicated by iris adhesions to the lens (posterior synechiae) or to the peripheral cornea (anterior synechiae) and secondary glaucoma.

Direct invasion of ocular tissue

This occurs in lepromatous disease and more often in temperate climates, producing a keratitis, scleritis and iritis.

Corneal disease

An asymptomatic fine punctate subepithelial infiltrate beginning in the upper temporal quadrant is the initial manifestation of involvement of the corneal nerve, which may become beaded and calcified due to aggregations of phagocytosed bacilli. Progression to other quadrants or deep stroma may occur but pannus is unusual unless accompanied by limbal granulomata.

A sclerokeratitis may be associated with leprous episcleritis or scleritis, while band keratopathy is a common feature of chronic iritis.

Uveal disease

While acute iritis may occur in all forms of leprosy, chronic iritis is limited to the lepromatous form in which there is a heavy bacillary invasion of the anterior uvea, whose temperature is some 3° less than body temperature, and contains numerous non-myelinated autonomic nerve fibres—the ideal conditions for multiplication.

Insidiously progressive, the mild iritis is associated in its early stages with discrete yellow globular deposits within the iris stroma (iris pearls), that gradually protrude and eventually fall into the anterior chamber—these are aggregates of phagocytosed bacilli within mononuclear cells.

With time, there is progressive iris atrophy, marked miosis and little response to cycloplegic drugs. This miosis in combination with axial corneal or lens opacities contributes greatly to the visual handicap and appears to be the result of preferential involvement of the dilator muscles. Posterior synechiae are not a feature of this neuroparalytic iritis but a flocculent inflammatory membrane may occlude the pupil, inducing pupil block glaucoma.

Management

The principal aim in management is the interruption of the cycle of transmission by using drugs such as the sulphones, which are bacteriostatic and to which there is increasing resistance, or the more expensive but bactericidal rifampicin.

But this aim is thwarted by the social stigma that accompanies this disease, a social prejudice against patients identified by limb and facial deformities. This has three main effects:

1   Patients become outcasts in their own communities.
2   Patients are reluctant to seek advice for fear of a diagnosis of leprosy and thus often present late in the disease with established neurological deficit.
3   In many countries medical and paramedical personnel are reluctant to treat leprosy.

Thus, education of lay and medical personnel about the true implications of leprosy is of prime importance.

Early identification of patients, within the context of primary health care, should be followed by regular surveillance of their families for signs of early leprosy—especially the punctate keratitis.

While the acute iritis is treated with mydriatics and steroids, it is doubtful that topical steroids, particularly with their ocular hypertensive and cataractogenic properties, are of any value in chronic iritis, but pupil dilatation using sympathomimetic drugs such as phenylephrine may be of benefit in preventing the incapacitating miosis.

The lid deformities require plastic surgical repair, and tear supplements. If there is impaired corneal sensation, the patient and his relatives are instructed to examine the eye daily for evidence of trauma or infection—impaired vision or redness of the eye—and if present to attend for medical advice.

Leprosy is an eminently treatable disease. Many patients do not receive treatment because of social prejudice. The challenge, therefore, is to overcome this stigma, to achieve earlier diagnosis and earlier treament and thus prevent deformity and blindness.

16

Hereditary Eye Diseases

C I Phillips

The objective of this chapter is *not* to impose on the student lists of rare diseases with their mode of inheritance but rather to use hereditary ophthalmic diseases to emphasize some simple basic principles used by geneticists in their clinics. The ophthalmological examples can easily be replaced by diseases from any or all specialties.

Hereditary eye disease is probably becoming more important as we are controlling more efficiently infections and other more environmental diseases, such as retrolental fibroplasia. In a school for the blind, around 50% of the pupils had definite evidence of a hereditary cause [1].

The clinician dealing with a suspected hereditary disease should be even more inclined to consult the literature than in ordinary clinical practice. An excellent starting point is McKusick's *Mendelian Inheritance in Man* [2].

Autosomal recessive inheritance is often missed [3]

Typical case: congenital retinal aplasia (Leber's congenital amaurosis)

Mrs B suspected that her daughter Fiona, aged $2\frac{1}{2}$ years, was blind. After a week of in-patient investigations it was confirmed that she probably had permanently poor vision but no other information was given. A second pregnancy produced a second daughter: by the time Marjorie was 6 months old, Mrs B was sure that her second child was also, tragically, blind. She then asked for genetic counselling and was told that 'congenital retinal aplasia' (Leber's congenital amaurosis) was not uncommon, and well known to be due to autosomal recessive genes. The risk to *any* future siblings would be 1 in 4 (Figs 16.1 and 16.2), which Mrs B and her husband decided was too great to take. She was sterilized.

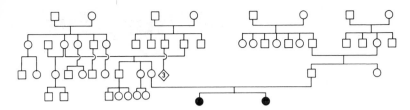

Fig 16.1 Congenital retinal aplasia ●, a not uncommon cause of blindness from birth or from an early age. Note the horizontal pattern in the family tree—i.e. only one generation affected, typical of autosomal recessive inheritance.

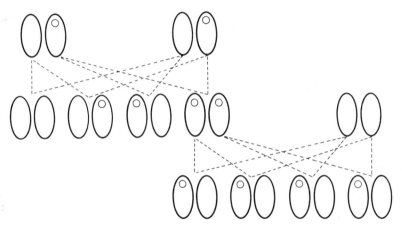

Fig 16.2 Autosomal recessive transmission. Top row: a pair of chromosomes 00 in a father (left) and mother (right). A small circle ○ indicates an autosomal recessive gene. Each parent is an unaffected carrier (heterozygous state) because a normal gene exists on the other chromosome. One in 4 of their children (second row) will have both recessive genes (the homozygous state) and so will suffer from the disease. The next generation (third row) is very unlikely to show the disease, even the children of the affected individual who is shown married to a normal spouse: in that case all the children will be carriers but unaffected. A warning against cousin marriages in such families is appropriate.

Examination of an affected baby's fundi (under general anaesthesia) shows little abnormality—pale discs and thin retinal arteries, but the normal baby's optic discs are pale. By the mid-teens the fundi usually show some pigmentary mottling in the mid-periphery, as in an early case of retinitis pigmentosa (*see* Plate 16.1). The electroretinogram is valuable in such cases and shows a poor or absent response to flashes of light; as would be expected, the visual evoked response (from the occipital cortex) is also poor.

An important clue to autosomal recessive genes as a cause for any disease is consanguinity of parents. When taking any family history, never omit to ask specifically if the parents are cousins, close or remote.

The sufferer from a disease due to the homozygous state of autosomal recessive genes (Figs 16.1 and 16.2) is very unlikely to pass on his disease to any children (provided the spouse is not a cousin: they should be specifically warned about that) because the gene frequency in the general population is usually low (Fig 16.2). Accordingly, the family tree in this mode of interitance is almost diagnostic at a glance: it has a **horizontal** pattern—i.e. only one generation is affected, all previous and subsequent generations being free from the disease (Figs. 16.1 and 16.2).

When *two* members of *one* generation have an identical, bilaterally symmetrical, eye disease, the autosomal recessive 'diagnosis' is usually fairly obvious, although other possible causes must be considered: however, a germ line mutation is a very unlikely possibility. Sporadic *single* cases—quite unexpected by the family—of appropriate diseases (e.g. retinitis pigmentosa, *see* below) are more common and often due to autosomal recessive genes, but the possibility of a dominant mutation or an environmental cause has to be considered more seriously than when more than one in a sibship are affected.

Autosomal dominant inheritance

This can also be diagnosed almost at a glance by inspecting the family tree. It shows a **vertical** pattern—i.e. the disease occurs in two or more generations (*see* Fig 16.4). The most important proviso is that you must check carefully that there are examples of male-to-male transmission in the family tree: if there is none, you must then consider X-linked recessive transmission (*see* below).

A typical family affected by dominant congenital cataract is shown in Fig 16.3. Presumably the first affected in that family represents a mutation to a dominant gene which has then been passed on to subsequent generations: without the evidence of subsequent generations, that first 'sporadic' case might well have been attributed to autosomal recessive genes or, as actually happened, might have been attributable to an intrauterine infection by the virus of rubella (German measles). Because rubella infection *can* cause congenital cataracts, deafness and/or heart disease, any of these conditions tends to be attributed to that infection, often wrongly—and turns out subsequently to be due to hereditary disease, either because a second sibling is affected or because a future generation is affected.

Figure 16.4 explains how the risk to a child is 50% at each pregnancy

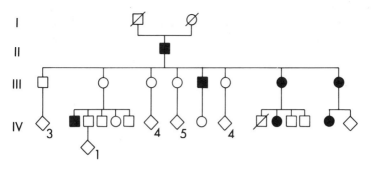

Fig 16.3 Dominant pattern of inheritance of congenital cataracts. Note the vertical pattern of the family tree: three generations are affected, one example of male-to-male transmission ■ and an apparent example of 'skipping' of a generation—i.e. in generation III the second child, a female, appears unaffected (○) but has an affected son. However, she had subclinical lens abnormalities visible with the slit-lamp microscope. The 'sporadic' case, a male in the first affected generation, presumptively represents a dominant mutation.

Key: ■ ● = male and female affected; □○ male and female unaffected; ◇ male and/or female unaffected.

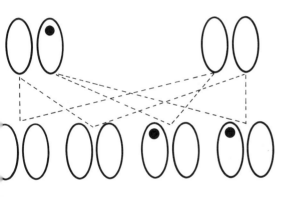

Fig 16.4 Autosomal dominant transmission. A pair of chromosomes 00 in a father (left) and mother (right). The small black circle ● indicates a dominant abnormal gene which overcomes the normal gene in its paired chromosome. A dominant disease affects the father. In the second generation (second row), 50% of the children can be expected to inherit the disease.

for a dominant disease, no matter whether the previous child is, or is not, affected. Patients understand very easily that even if the risk is 50% each time, the whole of a small (two or three) family may be all affected or all unaffected: they know that, over all, about 50% of the population are female and 50% are male but there are many sibships with only males or only females—i.e. the variance in small samples can be large.

X-linked recessive

X-linked recessive disease has a very characteristic pattern of family tree: males are affected and females are carriers. **Male-to-male transmission**

never occurs (save in the rarest exceptional circumstances such as in chromosome abnormalities) (*see* Figs 16.6 and 16.7).

Retinitis pigmentosa (primary pigmentary degeneration of the retina) is quite often inherited in this way. However, this clinical condition may be inherited in the autosomal recessive pattern (with slightly earlier onset and faster progression than in the X-linked form) or in a dominant pattern (with usually much later onset and slower progression). Therefore the disease is *not* a single entity—i.e. it must have several different (biochemical) causes. It is a bilaterally symmetrical disease with almost pathognomonic ophthalmoscopic appearances (*see* Plate 16.1). The patient first notices more difficulty than the normal has in seeing in very dull illumination ('night blindness'), then his fields of vision become progressively constricted from the periphery inwards until he can see only in the central area ('tunnel vision' or 'tube fields') (Fig 16.5).

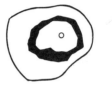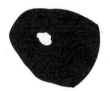

Fig 16.5 Fields of vision in retinitis pigmentosa. The left diagram (a left eye) shows an irregular black ring indicating a blind area (scotoma) in the mid-periphery of the field of vision: the small circle indicates the centre of the field. As the disease progresses, the scotoma extends peripherally and centrally until only a small central area of field (right diagram, a right eye) remains: 'tunnel vision' or 'tube field'. Both eyes are usually equally affected and progress equally.

Finally, complete blindness ensues after many years of increasing disability. No treatment will retard the progression of the disease, but magnifying spectacles and removal of the commonly complicating cataract can help considerably.

A typical family tree is shown in Fig 16.7; Fig 16.6 explains the mechanism.

It is a fascinating property of the X-linked form of this disease, like Duchenne muscular dystrophy and haemophilia, that the female carrier suffers from a variable but milder form of the disease which affects the male representative severely. This is because, very early in development, one X chromosome in each cell is suppressed at random: those in which the X chromosome containing the normal gene is suppressed will ultimately produce retinal cells suffering from retinitis pigmentosa

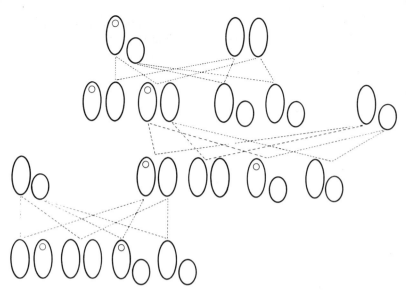

Fig 16.6 X-linked recessive transmission. Top row: a recessive gene ○ is present in the unpaired portion of the X chromosome of the father. The Y chromosome is smaller, and also has an unpaired portion (extending below the level of the lower end of the X). In the second row, all the daughters are carriers but all the sons escape the disease because they must have inherited their father's Y chromosome. A carrier daughter in the second row is shown married to a normal male: 50% of her sons will be affected and 50% of her daughters will be carriers. Another carrier daughter (third row) is shown married to a normal man: there is a 50% risk to any male child. Accordingly, an affected father has a 50% risk of having affected grandsons produced by his daughters.

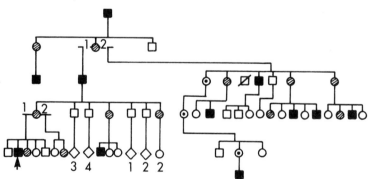

Fig 16.7 X-linked recessive retinitis pigmentosa. *Note the absence of any example of male-to-male transmission.* Males are severely and quickly progressively affected in early life ■, and go to blind schools and blind workshops. Females are variably affected, later in life ◕, because of suppression of one X chromosome at random at a very early stage in development, i.e. only a proportion of retinal cells will ultimately suffer from retinitis pigmentosa—only those in which the normal X chromosome is suppressed. Full details of females ⊙ were not available but they must have been carriers. The symbol ◇ means male or female, the figure attached indicating the number of siblings.

whereas those in which the other chromosome, containing the abnormal gene, is suppressed will ultimately form normal retinal cells [4]. The severity of the disease in the carrier female is very variable—usually mild, surprisingly (see Fig 16.7). The Barr body in female white blood cells represents the suppressed X chromosome. Accordingly, the female carrier's retina may show some peripheral pigmentation, with diminution in the flash-response in the electroretinogram and some abnormality in the dark adaptation curve.

Other hereditary eye diseases

Many diseases do not conform to a simple Mendelian pattern. As in vascular hypertension, the first-degree relatives of patients with glaucoma (open-angle or angle-closure glaucoma) have a higher risk than in the normal of having the disease. In these two glaucomas the risk is three to four times greater than usual, which suggests that screening of these relatives over the age of, say, 50 years may be worth doing.

The hereditary pattern in refractive errors, especially myopia, is not clear.

References

1 Phillips C I, Stokoe N L and Hughes Helen E. (1975) An ophthalmic genetics clinic. *Trans Ophthalmol Soc UK* **95**, 472–6
2 McKusick V A (1978) *Mendelian Inheritance in Man*, 5th edn. Baltimore and London: Johns Hopkins University Press
3 Phillips C I and Newton Marjorie S (1981) Beware recessive genes. *Lancet* **2**, 293–8
4 Lyon Mary (1962) Sex chromatin and gene action in the mammalian X chromosome. *Am J Hum Genet* **14**, 135–48

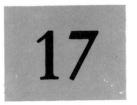

Some Preventive and Social Aspects

A R Elkington

The expression 'prevention is better than cure' is particularly relevant to those involved in preserving people's eyesight. One only has to think of the eradication of smallpox or the control of the fly vector of onchocerciasis in Kenya to appreciate that a preventive approach has saved millions of people from blindness [1]. Such preventive programmes can be successfully implemented only if the social customs both of the community and of individuals are thoroughly appreciated. And so it is right that preventive and social aspects are dealt with together. The need to think in these terms will already be apparent to the reader of many of the earlier chapters, particularly that on tropical diseases.

We should never forget the scale of the problem of worldwide blindness. It has been estimated that there are more than 40 million people in the world who are blind and perhaps 30 million of these are needlessly blind from a preventable cause. Such statements immediately raise the problem of defining blindness [2]. There are over 60 different definitions worldwide. The World Health Organization has advocated a general concept of visual impairment which is based on a relatively liberal scale which extends from an acuity of 6/24 to that of no perception of light. However, in the UK, for instance, the limits are more stringent. Someone in the UK is eligible for blind registration only 'if he cannot perform work for which eyesight is essential'. This usually means an acuity of 3/60 or less in the better eye or a much reduced visual field or both.

The need to register a patient blind should cause us to ask ourselves if the blindness could have been prevented. Let us look therefore, even if in a necessarily highly selective way, at how some forms of blindness can be prevented. Let us start at the beginning.

Pregnancy

To date we have but little understanding of the cause of most congenital abnormalities, many of which involve the visual pathways. (Remember, if you detect one congenital anomaly then look for others, because such abnormalities are commonly multiple.) One known cause of congenital malformations is rubella infection in the first trimester of pregnancy which may lead to the classic triad of cataracts, deafness and cardiac defects. The immunization of women of child-bearing age and selective abortion are preventive measures which have many social consequences. Then there is syphilis which can affect the fetus (and its eyes) in so many ways. The tracing of contacts and the proper treatment of infected persons should be vigorously pursued. And the thalidomide disaster should make all doctors wary of prescribing any drug to a woman who is, or might be, pregnant [3].

Birth and the neonatal period

Our entry into the world is fraught with hazard. The major risk is from anoxia, either during birth itself or in the first few days of life. Such anoxia may cause irreparable brain damage which may result in greatly impaired vision. The premature infant is particularly ill-equipped to survive the rigours of parturition, and often respiratory problems mean that the infant's hold on life is tenuous. The baby may be kept alive only by the administration of oxygen, which brings its own risks. The immature retinal vessels, particularly those in the temporal periphery, go into spasm when exposed to a high oxygen tension and tend to proliferate when the oxygen level is reduced (*see* Chapter 1). The proliferating vessels may invade the anterior part of the vitreous cavity and become progressively organized to form a mass of fibrous tissue behind the lens (retrolental fibroplasia). The earliest changes of this retinopathy of prematurity resolve in most cases, but once fibrous tissue is laid down there is a chance, perhaps years later, that its contraction will cause traction on the retina which may lead to retinal detachment. The paediatrician is thus caught between Scylla and Charybdis: too little oxygen and the baby dies; too much and it lives, but it may go blind.

Childhood

A youngster's eyesight is primarily at risk from a squint, an uncorrected refractive error or trauma.

Squint

Children born prematurely or those whose birth was difficult are particularly likely to develop a squint. So, too, are those who have relatives with a history of squint. These children should therefore be identified and screened with especial care. Attention should always be paid to what the mothers says about the child's eyes. (She is with her baby most of the time; we may have only a few moments to examine the child, who may be sleeping or fractious.) The proper way of carrying out the cover test should be learned, and regularly practised, by all those with the responsibility and opportunity of checking children's eyes.

Arrangements should be made for health visitors, and others concerned, to visit an orthoptic department for the necessary instruction. It should be stressed how important the test is, for failure to detect a squint may lead to a child's growing up with a densely amblyopic eye and if, in later life, through an accident or perhaps a vascular occlusion, the sight of the other eye is lost then the patient will be effectively blind. But the test is not always easy to carry out and instructors should be sympathetic towards trainees' difficulties.

Uncorrected refractive errors

The child who has a marked refractive error affecting both eyes has difficulty seeing clearly (only in the distance in the case of myopia) and the parents usually spot that there is something amiss and seek advice. In the case of the child with a unilateral refractive error (provided the acuity of the other eye is good) the error is likely to go undetected for some time, for children characteristically do not complain when they see poorly with one eye alone. The child with unilateral low myopia does not develop amblyopia because near objects are seen clearly with the abnormal eye, even if distant objects are blurred. But a highly myopic eye will become amblyopic. More commonly and typically, children with marked degrees of unilateral hypermetropia and astigmatism also develop amblyopia, for in each case the retinal image is constantly blurred.

The so-called 'straight-eyed amblyope' (i.e. anisometropic amblyope) is picked up only if the acuity of the two eyes is checked individually and this means that eyesight tests must be done properly. Sadly this is often not the case. Children peep between the fingers of the hand occluding their good eye and so seem to see perfectly well with their bad one. The school teachers, who so frequently take on these tests with considerable reluctance, should cover each eye in turn with a card to prevent such deception.

Trauma

A young child with a perforating eye injury in the arms of a weeping guilt-ridden young mother makes a very pathetic sight. Scissors, broken tableware, darts, fireworks and airgun pellets are regular culprits. Even the children of prudent parents grow up in a dangerous environment. That's life. But it behoves both parents and doctors to anticipate trouble and supervise potentially dangerous activities. Should a mishap occur then we should take a careful history (beware of the young member of a gang who is trying to cover up for his mates), carry out a thorough examination suspecting that there might be something wrong, and remember to think an x-ray which may reveal a retained foreign body.

The problem of non-accidental injury (the 'battered baby') is being increasingly recognized. Children may have bruising around the eye or have retinal haemorrhages or more extensive ocular damage. The suspicious clinician should enquire about any other hospital visits and look for other signs of injury which may be in various stages of resolution.

Young adult

Even in our prime our eyes are at risk. There are hazards both at work and at play. For those who come from a family with a hereditary eye disorder there will be the need to seek specialist advice before they embark upon either marriage or having children.

At work

The proper protection of the eye by means of spectacles with toughened lenses, or goggles or visors is all part and parcel of many jobs in modern industry. The design of these forms of protection should ensure not only that the eye is properly shielded but also that these devices are acceptable to the wearer. If lenses steam up or cumbersome headgear causes unbearable stuffiness, these protective measures will be discarded. Then there is the need to educate employees about caring for themselves and for one another. In factories where dangerous chemicals are used, every employee should know how to wash out an eye and be aware that speed in doing so is all-important.

Driving is a necessary part of many jobs. The visual requirements in the UK for driving a car are an acuity of 6/15 or better in at least one eye and an 'adequate' field of vision. The requirements to drive either a lorry (heavy goods vehicle) or a bus (public service vehicle) are stricter. Car drivers who become aware of a change in their eyesight which they feel may influence their ability to drive are duty bound to contact the licensing authority. Those patients who suddenly lose the sight of an eye should be warned not to drive until they have adapted to their new predicament. As might be expected, young people adapt quickly (in a few weeks) whilst older people take far longer and sometimes they never acquire sufficient confidence to drive again.

Shattered windscreens have accounted for many eyes being lost. Two measures should help to reduce this toll: first, the wearing of seat belts, which reduces the risk of the wearer being thrown forwards on to any remaining jagged fragments of glass; and, second, the use of laminated rather than toughened glass windscreens. The former crack but do not produce loose fragments of glass; it is rare for anything to go through such windscreens. The latter windscreens shatter into thousands of pieces and may thus cause extensive damage to both the face and the eyes.

At play

For many people, working hours are becoming shorter, which leaves more time for leisure pursuits. Badminton and squash are increasingly popular games and the shuttlecock and squash ball are small enough to pass within the rim of the orbit and so compress the eye: a well-struck squash ball travels at over 120 mph. The designers of the faceguards worn by ice hockey players whose efforts have led to such a dramatic reduction in the number of eye injuries in that game, are now turning their attention to squash in particular, and the use of eyeguards on the squash court is likely to become more common in the future.

Genetic counselling

People who are aware that there is an eye disease running through their family usually want to know what chance there is of passing it on to their children. Advice should be sought from a clinician particularly interested in such problems working in conjunction with a geneticist in a special clinic, for it is only in such a setting that the proper expertise can be developed and the many pitfalls of interpreting hereditary patterns be avoided. The marriage of two people who are blind may raise particularly difficult moral issues, for the chance of their children being blind may be very high indeed [4]. It is not surprising that those in blind homes should tend to marry others who are blind, not only because they are necessarily often segregated together but also because they share a similar affliction.

Those who have been blind from birth seem to underestimate the importance of eyesight: they have a different view to that of most of us on the risk of producing a blind child.

Middle age

The first clue for many people that the years are slipping by is the need to take to reading glasses. The progressive loss of the ability to accommodate means that most Caucasians require a presbyopic correction at about the age of 45 years (those from the Indian subcontinent usually need reading glasses five years earlier). In some parts of the world such glasses can be chosen in a bazaar on a trial-and-error basis, but a better arrangement would be for a refraction to be carried out which would allow a more precise prescription to be provided, thus enabling the wearer to see as well as possible. Such an examination would ideally also allow scrutiny of the eyes; some disorders (notably chronic open-angle glaucoma) are often detected in this way.

Refractions are carried out in the UK by a variety of practitioners. Most of the 400 or so consultant ophthalmologists practise privately part-time, and perform refractions in their consulting rooms. Then there are about 600 ophthalmologists who work partly as clinical assistants in hospital eye departments and also as ophthalmic medical practitioners (OMPs) at medical eye centres (MECs). These centres are usually adjacent to the premises of one of the 2000 dispensing opticians (DOs) in the country who do not themselves refract but who make up glasses to someone else's prescription. However, the bulk of refractions are carried out by the 6000 ophthalmic opticians (OOs) who work from separate premises. Most ophthalmic opticians do their own dispensing, for there is more money to be made from selling glasses than from the examination fee. Opticians of both varieties work either in an individual practice or as part of a firm (or multiple) which may have many branches throughout the country.

The middle years may see the onset of a disease for which drugs are prescribed. Rheumatoid arthritis may be treated with hydroxychloroquine, which is taken up selectively by the retinal pigment epithelium which may, in turn, lead to macular damage. A total cumulative dose of 800 g should not be exceeded [5]. The same condition (and many others) may be treated with systemic steroids, which may lead to the development of opacities at the posterior pole of the lens. These opacities lie close to the nodal point of the eye where they particularly interfere with vision. A host of inflammatory disorders are treated with steroid eyedrops; some people develop a marked rise in intraocular pressure when such drops are used (the so-called 'steroid responders') and glaucoma, with resulting blindness, can be induced. Patients who have been prescribed topical steroids should therefore have their intraocular pressure checked regularly. Many other drugs affect the eye, and the prescribing doctor should always bear this in mind.

Old age

This is when degenerative disorders set in and it is only rarely that these processes can be arrested. However, the visual consequences of these disorders can often be mitigated.

Cararact

The use of the word itself causes many old people great anxiety. They may remember an elderly relative being blind after a cataract operation that 'went wrong'. When only slight lens opacities are detected it is better to use a term such as 'cloudiness of the lens' rather than talk about a cataract, for the opacities may not change during the few remaining years left to the patient and, by use of the former term, needless anxiety can be avoided. Should operation become advisable and the word 'cataract' be used then it should be pointed out that surgery these days is much safer than it used to be.

Surgeons who enjoy removing cataracts may find giving advice about lighting rather tedious. But to the patient such mundane advice may be an enormous boon and enable him to read once again. A lamp with a 100 watt bulb should be placed behind the patient so that the light is thrown directly on to the page. This is far preferable to the all too common arrangement of a 60 watt bulb dangling from a flex set in the middle of the ceiling. If the patient is having difficulty from loss of field due to a unilateral cataract then advice about turning his head to that side can make life much easier for him. The same holds true for those patients with a homonymous hemianopia.

Macular degeneration

Most patients with this condition notice increasing difficulty with the vision of both eyes and they are terrified that they are eventually going to go completely blind. They rarely express this fear but its intensity is betrayed by the sigh of relief that they let out when it is explained to them that there is no question of their going truly blind. Because the peripheral retina remains healthy, peripheral and hence navigational vision is retained. The patients will be able to get about their homes and do indoor chores. They will be able to dress and feed themselves. They will probably always see enough to go outside alone, although they will need help crossing roads and when in unfamiliar surroundings. They will not be able to recognize faces at a distance or see the numbers of approaching buses. Shopkeepers may well need to take their purses to count out the change. Signing pension books may only be possible if someone shows them where to write: this is best done by placing the forefinger of the patient's free hand at the beginning of the line. But despite all these inconveniences they will not go blind. It is important to 'test' these patients' fields to confrontation in order to demonstrate to them that their peripheral fields are full.

Patients with macular degeneration often see much better if they are provided with some form of magnifying device or 'low vision aid'. The benefit derived from any of these aids depends upon the fact that the retina surrounding the macula is healthy and if the retinal image is sufficiently enlarged then these paramacular areas can be used. A suitable telescope, for instance, may allow a patient to watch television; reading, too, may become possible again with the use of either a simple magnifying glass or some more sophisticated instrument. It should be remembered that with increasing magnification the field of view becomes smaller and the range of focus is progressively reduced. These factors may set such limitations that it may be impossible to help some patients by these means.

Glaucoma

This term is used to describe a group of ocular disorders in which the intraocular pressure is too high. There are many ways in which the pressure can become raised and so there are many forms of glaucoma. As a general rule if the pressure rises quickly then pain is induced but if the increase in pressure is gradual then the condition is likely to be pain-free. In the former event the person concerned usually seeks advice, but in the latter situation the glaucoma sufferer may be unaware of anything amiss and his eyesight may be severely affected by the time the glaucoma is diagnosed. The chronically raised intraocular pressure is associated with a specific type of optic atrophy (glaucomatous cupping of the optic disc) and characteristic field loss. In the early stages of the disease the blind areas (scotomata) lie adjacent to, but do not involve, the central field of vision. The acuity is unaffected and, indeed, this is often preserved right up to the time when all sight is finally lost. So, unlike virtually all other eye disorders, in chronic forms of glaucoma a good acuity may be retained in the face of gross ocular disease.

Open-angle glaucoma is the most important disease in this connection. It is relatively common, affecting in the UK 1 in 200 of those over 40 years of age. It usually affects both eyes, but often one more than the other. In view of its importance as a cause of blindness and because there may be no symptoms, various screening programmes have been set up to try to identify those with the disease at an early stage, when treatment often arrests further field loss. Such programmes have largely foundered for the following reasons. First, open-angle glaucoma can be neither diagnosed nor excluded on a pressure reading alone (*see* Chapter 5). Secondly, field estimation requires special equipment and is time-consuming. And thirdly, inspection of the optic disc (by far the best way of either incriminating or ruling out open-angle glaucoma) requires the skill of an experienced observer. These problems have led those responsible for organizing health care programmes to abandon such an all-encompassing approach as being not cost-effective. Accordingly, there is now great interest in identifying high-risk groups. For instance, it has been shown that first-degree relatives (siblings and children) of patients with open-angle glaucoma have a ten to fifteenfold chance of developing the disease when compared with members of the general population. This has led to family clinics being set up and some early cases are being detected in this way. The identification of these patients makes a welcome change from those who discover one eye is blind when, for some reason, they cover the other eye. And also a welcome change from those who are discovered to have gross pathological cupping of the discs at refraction or the patient who presents with occlusion of the central retinal vein—a well recognized complication of the glaucoma. Detecting the earliest signs of glaucomatous cupping of the disc is all-important, and all practitioners should aim to become competent at scrutinizing the nerve head. It is worth remembering that most of us have right and left optic discs that are remarkably alike. If the patient's discs look dissimilar then suspect glaucoma. But identifying the patient with glaucoma is not the end of the matter. Far from it. Regular supervision, with all the implications in terms of clinic time, will need to be arranged for the rest of the patient's life. And just because we write up treatment should not lead us to suppose that it is being taken. A recent study has shown that only half the patients interviewed were taking the medication as prescribed.

Welfare services for the blind

It will be clear from what has already been written that people's sight may be impaired for a whole variety of reasons. As the patient's vision worsens progressively it is appropriate that he receive increasing help from the supporting services. In the UK such support is triggered by the ophthalmologist's completing a form BD8, registering the patient as either partly sighted or blind. An acuity of 6/36 in both eyes, or a better acuity if there is extensive field loss, will allow partial registration. This ensures that the patient is known to the welfare services and that he is visited by a social worker who should co-ordinate the help from the community due to the patient. A low vision aid may be suggested and a 'talking-book' (a tape recorder with cassettes on which are recorded novels, biographies, etc.) may be provided. For children there are specially trained teachers, and for those of working age a range of rehabilitation programmes. For those registered blind the help is more comprehensive. They pay reduced fares if they travel to work. The licence for a guide dog is free and that for a television set reduced. Patients may be able to claim certain tax advantages. They have access to a mobility officer who is specially trained to advise patients how best to get about and look after themselves; this adviser is in a position to recommend those aids that make everyday tasks, such as cooking and using the telephone, much easier for those who cannot see. He will also instruct those people who spend time with the patient how to be of the greatest possible help. He will, for instance, point out that the best way of leading a blind patient about is to walk arm in arm slightly in front and to one side of him. In this way the patient gets clues about the environment from the movements the other person makes. A step down is appreciated before it is reached by the patient because the helper is felt to move down, and so on.

In this chapter we have done no more than explore some of the many ways in which eyesight may be preserved by our adopting an anticipatory approach to possible eye problems. It has surely become clear that such a preventive approach has all sorts of social implications which also have to be considered in evolving a practical attitude as to how preventable blindness may be avoided. After all, to be forewarned is to be forearmed.

References

1 Jones B R (1978) Prevention of blindness. What is it all about? *Trans Ophthalmol Soc UK* **98**, 282–6
2 Cullinan T R (1982) Blind ignorance. *Health Services* no. 32 (17 Sep), 12–13
3 Reynolds J E F (ed) (1982) *Martindale: the Extra Pharmacopoeia*, 27th edn. London: Pharmaceutical Press
4 Phillips C I, Newton M S and Gosden C M (1982) Procreative instinct as a contributory factor to prevalence of hereditary blindness. *Lancet* **1**, 1169–72
5 Mills P V, Beck M and Power B J (1981) Assessment of the retinal toxicity of hydroxychloroquine. *Trans Ophthalmol Soc UK* **101**, 109–13

Index